# Psychiatry Update 2

**Series Editor**
Michelle B. Riba
University of Michigan, Department of Psychiatry
University of Michigan Eisenberg Family Depression Center
Ann Arbor, MI, USA

Psychiatry Update will encompass all areas of psychiatry research and clinical diagnosis and treatment. Chapters will publish randomly though out the year culminating in volumes throughout the year.

More information about this series at http://www.springer.com/series/16222

Jonathan D. Avery • David Hankins
Editors

# Addiction Medicine

## A Case and Evidence-Based Guide

Springer

*Editors*
Jonathan D. Avery
Weill Cornell Medicine
NewYork-Presbyterian Hospital
New York, NY
USA

David Hankins
Weill Cornell Medicine
NewYork-Presbyterian Hospital
New York, NY
USA

ISSN 2524-8316 ISSN 2524-8324 (electronic)
Psychiatry Update 2
ISBN 978-3-030-86429-3 ISBN 978-3-030-86430-9 (eBook)
https://doi.org/10.1007/978-3-030-86430-9



This Springer imprint is published by the registered company Springer Nature Switzerland AG
The registered company address is: Gewerbestrasse 11, 6330 Cham, Switzerland

# Introduction by Series Editor

It is an honor to welcome this edited book by Drs. Avery, Hankins, et al. on addiction medicine to this series.

Substance use disorders and other mental health conditions are a growing problem, especially during the recent COVID pandemic. We are learning more and more about the interrelationship between the neurobiology of addiction, behavioral manifestations, co-occurrence with other psychiatric problems, and associated social, economic, and intergenerational issues.

Training in this specific field is a complicated but necessary part of mental health care, with growing numbers of healthcare professionals recognizing the need to equip students, residents, and fellows with the necessary tools for maintaining competence in addiction medicine treatment.

In this edited book, we are delighted to present, along with seasoned authors, residents and fellows who validate the interest and trajectory of trainees who want to specialize in this area. This book contributes to the shared goals of clinicians who wish to attain improved clinical knowledge and proficiency on various topics in addiction medicine.

As we see more states in the USA legalize or allow the use of substances for medicinal or recreational purposes, it is incumbent upon health-care providers to better understand how to prevent, educate, recognize, evaluate, and treat substance use problems in a timely manner; this is a public health matter and mandate.

We thank the many authors who have contributed to this volume and Dr. Avery and Dr. Hankins for their leadership in organizing such a clinically valuable and comprehensive text.

# Introduction

Medical providers regardless of specialty encounter the effects of substance use and other addictive disorders on a daily basis. These effects of addictive behaviors, both direct and indirect, are responsible for vast morbidity and mortality globally as well as significant economic costs. Attitudes about substance use are rapidly shifting, leading to massive public policy and legal changes at the local, state, and national levels. These broader consequences make the value of discussing addiction with individual patients clear, but those conversations can be challenging for many reasons. Patients may feel hesitant to discuss their substance use related to shame and pervasive stigma. Providers may not be confident in their knowledge and skill level with assessing these disorders and so may do so incompletely or not at all. And both provider and patient may feel uneasy in navigating treatment options once a substance use disorder diagnosis has been made.

Luckily, this book has been written at a time when treatment options for substance use disorders continue to expand. Novel pharmacologic approaches are emerging for a variety of disorders, and there continue to be many well-studied, evidence-based medications available for some substance use disorders that remain underutilized. Options for psychotherapy, group treatment, and other psychosocial interventions are expanding as the treatment of addiction becomes a higher priority for the medical system and policymakers. There are excellent treatment options available for substance use disorders, and a physician may be the first person a patient turns to for help in these cases.

This book attempts to counter some of the potential pitfalls in the clinical encounter by the use of clinical cases in addiction. It primarily follows the structure of the *Diagnostic and Statistical Manual of Mental Disorders, 5th Edition* (DSM 5), with each substance use disorder featured in one chapter which centers on a clinical vignette (or vignettes) and provides helpful background on the etiology and treatment options for each disorder. If you are looking for help with a specific patient or a specific kind of addiction, you can jump immediately to the chapter about that disorder. We have also included chapters on the assessment of substance use disorders, their neurobiology, behavioral addictions, and the management of co-occurring psychiatric and substance use disorders, to provide additional context to those who would like to explore these topics at greater depth.

The cases presented in the book are not the stories of individual, real patients. They are intended to be "typical" cases, however, so may share similarities with patients the authors and readers have encountered. The cases are a mixture of some elements of the histories of patients treated by the authors as well as fictionalized elements included to facilitate broader discussion of each disorder. The names chosen by the authors are unrelated to any real patients treated by them.

All of the chapter authors wish you much success as you broach these at times difficult – but often lifesaving – discussions with your patients.

# Contents

# Contributors

**Jonathan D. Avery, MD** Weill Cornell Medicine, NewYork–Presbyterian Hospital, New York, NY, USA

**Matthew Boyer, MD** Rogers Behavioral Health, Philadelphia, PA, USA

**Noel Carrillo, MD** Weill Cornell Medicine, NewYork-Presbyterian Hospital, New York, NY, USA

**Rosemary Busch Conn, MD** Weill Cornell Medicine, NewYork-Presbyterian Hospital, New York, NY, USA

**Emily Dumas, MD** Weill Cornell Medicine, NewYork-Presbyterian Hospital, New York, NY, USA

**Sierra Ferguson, MD** Icahn School of Medicine at Mount Sinai, Mount Sinai Health System, New York, NY, USA

**Manesh Gopaldas, MD** Vanderbilt University Medical Center, Nashville, TN, USA

**David Hankins, MD** Weill Cornell Medicine, NewYork-Presbyterian Hospital, New York, NY, USA

**Kristopher A. Kast, MD** Vanderbilt University School of Medicine, Addiction Consult Service, Vanderbilt University Medical Center, Nashville, TN, USA

**Katherine Kim, MD** New York University Grossman School of Medicine, New York, NY, USA

**Dhruti Patel, MD** University of Miami Miller School of Medicine, Miami, FL, USA

**Daniel Roberts, MD, MSW** New York University Grossman School of Medicine, New York, NY, USA

**Keriann Shalvoy, MD** New York University Grossman School of Medicine, New York, NY, USA

**Daniel Sugrue, MD** Weill Cornell Medicine, NewYork-Presbyterian Hospital, New York, NY, USA

**Kseniya Svyatets, DO** New York University Grossman School of Medicine, New York, NY, USA

**Aviva Teitelbaum, MD** New York University Grossman School of Medicine, New York, NY, USA

**Anil Abraham Thomas, MD** New York University Grossman School of Medicine, New York, NY, USA

# 1 Assessment of Substance Use Disorders

Anil Abraham Thomas and Keriann Shalvoy

Substance use disorders are complex, chronic, relapsing and remitting diseases resulting in significant morbidity and mortality. The assessment of a possible substance use disorder or disorders is a fluid process that is the continuation of a positive triage screen. The assessment should clarify the diagnosis, type and extent of the disorder and should help determine the appropriate level of care. The assessment should also identify comorbid medical and psychiatric issues and help determine appropriate treatments [1]. Substance use assessment should use multiple avenues to collect the necessary clinical information, including clinical records, self-assessment instruments, structured clinical interviews, and collateral information whenever possible [2, 3].

## Gathering the History

Patients should be assessed along three domains: the medical domain, the psychiatric domain, and the substance use domain. Objective assessment includes the initial screening, mental status exam, physical exam, and diagnostic tools including ordering necessary laboratory and imaging studies. The mental status and physical exams can indicate whether the patient is currently intoxicated or in withdrawal. Pertinent positives and negatives differ depending on the substance being used by the patient and are discussed in more detail in later chapters of this book. Similarly, screening and diagnostic scales as well as laboratory and imaging studies can also be tailored to the differential diagnosis.

Assessing a patient along a medical domain is important particularly since a number of medical conditions can mimic various stages of a substance use disorder from intoxication, to withdrawal, to chronic use. For example, essential tremor in a

A. A. Thomas (✉) · K. Shalvoy
New York University Grossman School of Medicine, New York, NY, USA
e-mail: anil.thomas@nyulangone.org



J. D. Avery, D. Hankins (eds.), *Addiction Medicine*, Psychiatry Update 2,
https://doi.org/10.1007/978-3-030-86430-9_1

social alcohol user can be mistaken for acute alcohol withdrawal, or a gait abnormality attributed to substance abuse and not a neurological issue, if a detailed assessment is not completed. Table 1.1 highlights a selection of medical issues that might present similarly to a substance use disorder; keep in mind that this table is not exhaustive and that contributions from medical and psychiatric issues, as well as substance use, often remain on the differential diagnosis without it being possible to firmly eliminate one. Medical assessment enables one to quantify the comorbid issues that can influence treatment; it also helps to determine the extent of any medical complications as a result of the substance use disorder [4, 5]. The reverse is also true—substance use disorders can also mimic or precipitate common medical conditions. Common examples include nasal ulcers or perforated septum, skin track marks, skin abscesses, alcohol on breath, ascites, enlarged liver, obesity, uncontrolled hypertension, chronic pain, blackouts, accidental overdose, withdrawal symptoms, premature labor, and vague somatic complaints [6].

Assessing along the psychiatric domain is equally important; here again there are psychiatric conditions that can mimic substance use disorders. For example, untreated anxiety might be mistaken for alcohol withdrawal or cocaine intoxication if the patient endorses any recent use of one of these substances, leading to a missed diagnosis of generalized anxiety disorder or panic disorder. As with medical issues, substance use disorders can also mimic common psychiatric conditions. Common symptoms that can be associated with a wide range of substance intoxication and withdrawal syndromes include depression, anxiety, paranoia, hallucinations, irritability, insomnia, flashbacks, suicidal ideations, vagueness, memory and concentration issues, and defensiveness when questioned about substance use. Brain imaging

**Table 1.1** Examples of medical "mimics" of substance use disorders and their complications

| | |
|---|---|
| Head, eyes, ears, nose, and throat (HEENT) | Rhinorrhea seen in patients with upper respiratory infections (similar to that seen in opioid withdrawal) |
| Cardiovascular | Palpitations seen in patients with atrial fibrillation with rapid ventricular response (similar to that seen with stimulant intoxication or alcohol withdrawal) |
| Respiratory | Shortness of breath seen in patients with coronavirus disease 2019 (COVID-19) (similar to that seen with chronic cigarette smoking) |
| Gastrointestinal | Vomiting seen in patients with acute appendicitis (similar to that seen with alcohol intoxication) |
| Genitourinary | Dysuria seen in patients with acute urinary tract infections (similar to that seen with chronic ketamine use) |
| Dermatologic | Facial and oral lesions seen in patients with fixed drug eruption (similar to those seen with inhalant abuse) |
| Neurologic | Gait disturbance and dysarthria seen in patients with posterior circulation stroke (similar to that seen with alcohol intoxication) |
| Endocrine | Diarrhea seen in patients with hyperthyroidism (similar to that seen in opioid withdrawal) |
| Hematologic | Paranoia seen in patients with acute intermittent porphyria (similar to that seen with methamphetamine intoxication) |
| Allergy/immunology | Conjunctival injection from allergic rhinitis (similar to that seen with cannabis use) |

of people who have substance use disorders has shown changes in areas responsible for decision-making, learning, memory, judgment, behavioral control, and overall body functioning, any one of which could also be attributed to a primary psychiatric issue in a certain context [7]. Screening for suicidal ideation and depression should be included in all substance-related disorder assessments, e.g., the Columbia Suicide Severity Rating Scale (C-SSRS) and the Patient Health Questionnaire-9 (PHQ-9) [8].

Fully considering medical and psychiatric issues potentially at play can help prevent premature closure and false attribution of symptoms to substance use alone, which can have serious consequences. However, a comprehensive assessment of substance use is always essential along with the other two domains. The substance use history should begin with open-ended questioning ("Have you ever used any substances, regularly or socially, including using prescription drugs that you don't get from a doctor or use differently or for longer periods than they are prescribed?") and move toward a systematic approach to specifically address each substance individually. Assessment of the substance use domain should determine all the substances the person uses, the extent or quantity of use for each substance (whether in money spent or other kinds of quantity data such as cigarettes smoked or bags of heroin used), the length of time of use for each substance including the timing of first lifetime use of the substance and last time the substance was used, the pattern of use (daily, binging, occasional, social, etc.), and the route of administration: oral, intranasal, smoking, intraocular, or intravenous. These questions and others can be thought of on a spectrum of urgency as illustrated in Table 1.2. Certain questions must be asked immediately to prevent life-threatening consequences, while other questions may be part of a more comprehensive assessment or longer-term treatment and can help assess the patient's relationship to substances and willingness to change.

It is helpful to discuss the social situations that might have predisposed, precipitated, and perpetuated the patient's substance use, given the link between psychosocial stressors (divorce, loss of employment, housing instability) and worsening substance abuse [4]. As much as possible, the assessment should also determine the patient's level of interest in engaging in treatment and any particular barriers (whether practical or psychological) that might interfere. This can include

**Table 1.2** Question domains for the substance use history sorted by urgency

| Facts needed immediately | Facts to gather during the assessment | Facts and feelings to gather eventually |
|---|---|---|
| • Substances used<br>• Frequency and amount used most recently<br>• Route of administration<br>• Exact time of last use<br>• Any history of complicated alcohol or benzodiazepine withdrawal | • Age of first use<br>• Changes in pattern of use<br>• Longest period of abstinence<br>• Treatment history<br>• Family history with substances<br>• History of overdoses | • Does patient see substance use as a problem<br>• Likes/dislikes about substance use<br>• Reasons to change<br>• Financial consequences<br>• Triggers for use/relapse and adaptive strategies that have worked in the past |

discussion of the longest period of sobriety and interventions that aided in sobriety, as well as the causes of relapse.

If a thorough substance history is obtained, commonly used screening tools such as the CAGE (felt you should **C**ut down on use; people **A**nnoyed you by criticizing your use; felt bad or **G**uilty about use; ever use first thing in the morning to steady nerves or to get rid of any early withdrawal—"**E**ye opener"), or other questionnaires that are directed toward primary care or general psychiatric interviews, will be unnecessary [9].

In most cases, a basic urine drug screen involving qualitative opiate, methadone, cocaine, benzodiazepine, and barbiturates is indicated. If additional substance use is suspected, by the initial assessment, further toxicology diagnostics should be ordered. Routine medical labs including complete blood count, basic metabolic panel, hepatic function panel, hemoglobin A1c, and thyroid-stimulating hormone/free T4 are also indicated and can be tailored to the differential diagnosis. All women of child-bearing age should be given a pregnancy test given the significant risk for complications in pregnant women with comorbid substance use disorders. For patients with higher-risk sexual behaviors, a sexually transmitted infections (STI) panel including human immunodeficiency virus (HIV) testing should be ordered. For patients who use intravenous drugs, HIV, hepatitis B, and hepatitis C serologies should also be obtained. Tuberculosis testing may be indicated if the patient has a history of untreated HIV or is at high risk of it because of social circumstances [10].

## Making a Substance Use Disorder Diagnosis

Subsequent to gathering and analyzing the information, a diagnosis must be formulated. Diagnosis of a substance use disorder follows the criteria set forth in the Diagnostic and Statistical Manual 5 (DSM 5), with these general diagnostic criteria applied across the board to each specific substance use disorders (Table 1.3). The diagnosis requires "a problematic pattern of substance use leading to clinically significant impairment or distress as manifested be at least two of the 11 criteria, occurring within a 12 month period" [11]. To clarify the diagnosis, one needs to incorporate questions that address the DSM 5 criteria for substance use disorders (Table 1.3).

Some patients may find reviewing these DSM-5 criteria directly helpful as part of shared decision-making; others may bristle at the clinical language or reject that any of them apply to the patient's specific situation. As always, clinical judgment of the individual patient is essential.

## Discussing Treatment Options

If you have made a determination that the patient is likely to meet criteria for a substance use disorder, it is important at the initial assessment to determine the patient's readiness to change. The stages of change include pre-contemplation (unaware or unwilling to change; in denial), contemplation (considering change; ambivalent about change), preparation (experimenting with small changes), action (definite action to change), maintenance (maintaining new behavior), and relapse prevention

**Table 1.3** DSM-5 criteria for substance use disorder [11]

| | |
|---|---|
| At least two criteria occurring within a 12-month period | |
| 1 | Social and interpersonal problems |
| 2 | Craving or strong desire to use |
| 3 | Use in physically hazardous situations |
| 4 | Failure to fulfill major role obligations |
| 5 | Use larger amounts or for longer periods than intended |
| 6 | Desire or unsuccessful efforts to cut down |
| 7 | Important social, occupational, and recreational activities given up or reduced |
| 8 | Greater time spent to obtain, use, and recover |
| 9 | Use despite persistent or recurrent physical and psychological problems |
| 10 | Tolerance |
| 11 | Withdrawal |
| | Severity modifier: |
| | Mild: 2–3 criteria |
| | Moderate: 4–5 criteria |
| | Severe: 6 or more criteria |

[12, 13]. These stages for most are gradual, and it is expected that the patient will make advances and at times regress. One should also determine the positive and negative impact on the patient's quality of life; this includes understanding why using the substance is positively reinforcing for the patient or what benefits it provides [10, 14]. Working to understand the perceived positive aspects of substance use can help reduce feelings of judgment and stigma that the patient may have experienced in previous clinical encounters and may facilitate a fuller discussion of the more negative aspects of the substance use.

Discussion about treatment options must be handled carefully, as it requires the patient to have some understanding and agreement that there is a substance use disorder diagnosis at play. Prematurely discussing future treatment options with patients who do not have insight into having a substance use disorder (e.g., those at the pre-contemplation stage) may cause these patients to become angry and to stop engaging with the assessment.

## Common Challenges in the Substance Use Assessment

All substance use assessments should be informed by the possibility that patients may be acutely intoxicated or in withdrawal, influencing their ability or willingness to engage in a discussion. A patient who is intoxicated on phencyclidine (PCP) may be too agitated to participate in any sort of meaningful discussion; a patient who is withdrawing from heroin may become irritated if the conversation lasts too long and veers into less immediately relevant territory.

All conversations with the patient should be direct, empathic, and nonjudgmental in order to present information without alienating the patient who may be ashamed, in denial, ambivalent, or resistant to change. The approach can have a significant impact on whether the patient will leave the assessment in a position to take the next step forward [10].

All aspects of gathering a substance use history must be informed by the fact that patients often are reluctant to reveal substance use issues. There is a fear of negative judgment, being embarrassed by their inability to control their lives, or denial about the extent of the problem. These are the norm, not the exception. Patients avoid disclosing information in a variety of ways both subtle and more overt: minimizing use, minimizing consequences of use, changing topics, seeming not to listen, or discouraging questions with irritation and at times lying. The dropout rate within 30 days of initial assessment across substance use disorders is approximately 50%, with estimates ranging from 26% to 80% [15].

Providers should also be aware of how their own negative views of people who use substances—not always overt but often subtly informed by personal experiences and messages from superiors during medical training—may be affecting the quality of their relationship with the patient in the initial assessment. These biases toward patients with substance use disorders have the potential to negatively affect the likelihood of successful treatment. Physicians have higher rates of stigma toward substance-related disorders as compared to other illness, as well as pessimism about the role of treatment, which leads to decreased empathy toward patients with substance-related disorders [16].

Using multiple substances is common, although the patient may only view one as problematic. A patient who is perfectly content to discuss his significant daily use of intravenous heroin may angrily shut down any discussion of smoking cessation. Bearing in mind that a single patient's readiness to change on two different substances can be drastically different can help avoid an approach that damages the therapeutic alliance.

The involvement of family, friends, and previous providers can be useful in clarifying the patient's history and can be an essential part of a patient making the decision to begin treatment. When gathering collateral information or involving social supports in other ways, it is important to maintain the patient's trust and autonomy by obtaining written consent. You should encourage collateral information sources to share the extent of what they know about the patient's substance use, since patients themselves may be unreliable historians. Bringing support into the assessment whether by phone, video, or in person can be helpful in understanding the full extent of substance use. For example, patients may admit to more problematic aspects of substance use when directly confronted by a family member in ways that a provider cannot do. This can also be an opportunity to assess the family or other social support structures and the ways in which these could be beneficial in planning for next steps in treatment.

Finally, frequent reassessment is critical given the natural course of substance use disorders. The complexity and idiosyncratic features of substance withdrawal, cravings for the substance, and lingering chronic effects of long-time use are among the many factors that can make recovery from substance use so challenging and the presentation so varied at different points even for the same patient. Treatment adjustment is essential as needs of the patient evolve.

## Case Study: Patient Lilly

This patient case highlights some of the key considerations for substance use assessment discussed in this chapter.

History of Present Illness (HPI): 42-year-old woman in the emergency department (ED) requesting treatment for anxiety, insomnia, and methadone for withdrawal from heroin use. Patient indicates she "is tired of using and wants to change."

Medical Domain: Patient reports a diagnosis of hepatitis C for which she is not currently in treatment. She is vague about how she acquired it. She has a history of long-standing hypertension for which she is not in treatment, as well as psoriasis with flare-ups when stressed.

Psychiatric Domain: Patient complains of anxiety which is described as being continuous. She struggles to identify specific domains of anxiety, describing a much more generalized feeling of unease. She also complains of insomnia; she states she only sleeps for a "few hours" a day, and she is continuously tired. She denied any suicidal ideation currently (C-SSRS score is 0), and she denied any history of any suicide attempts. She has not followed up with a mental health professional.

Substance Use Domain: Opioids: heroin, using intravenously, currently using about 15 "bags" per day (equivalent to about 1.5 g per day although the amount of heroin per bag can vary in different communities). First opioid use at the age of 25 years—prescription pills after wisdom tooth removal—transitioned to using heroin at the age of 28. Last use was night prior to ED visit at around 10 pm, used 10 "bags" IV. She reports two prior accidental overdoses both requiring naloxone use and hospital stay. She denies any medical complications including endocarditis; however as noted she reports a history of hepatitis C. She has had multiple attempts at cutting down the use of heroin, by herself and also in treatment programs including two methadone maintenance program admissions. Longest period of sobriety since initial use of opioids was 2.5 years while in the methadone program, ending 1 year ago. Cocaine: ~$50 per day (~0.5 g), IV-"speedballs" (IV cocaine and heroin together), and first use was at the age of 26 and last use was night prior to ED visit, unknown amount. Tobacco: smokes one pack of cigarettes per day for the last 25 years. Denies use of other substances.

Family History: Patient denies any significant history; however she is vague about this.

Social History: She states she was born and raised in New York City, undomiciled, no contact with parents or siblings who also live in New York City. Not in any relationship. She has some college level education, no vocational training. She works odd jobs at times currently and has a history of sex work. She admits to a pending court case for shoplifting and has spent a total of 4 years in prison. No history of military service.

Objective Diagnostics: Positive urine toxicology for opioids and cocaine; positive serology for hepatitis C. Negative pregnancy test, negative HIV, mild elevation of transaminases.

Physical Exam: Suboptimal hygiene and grooming, cachectic, "track marks" secondary to IV drug use present on both arms and hands, chronic cough, and mildly elevated blood pressure.

Mental Status Exam (MSE): Most notable for superficially cooperative attitude, at times vague thought process, mild subjective anxiety, no hallucinations/delusions, no suicidal ideation currently, partial insight, impaired judgment.

Discussion: Patient Lilly came to the emergency department for anxiety, insomnia, and opioid withdrawal. It quickly becomes clear that she meets DSM-5 criteria for opioid use disorder, severe. She also likely meets criteria for cocaine use disorder, severe (under the category of stimulant use disorders), and tobacco use disorder, severe. The chronic nature of her medical and psychiatric issues raises the possibility of some significant contribution from either or both of these domains to her current presentation. For example, she may have any number of undiagnosed medical conditions exacerbating her insomnia and anxiety, particularly in light of her lack of engagement in medical care. Patients with chronic mental illness often have co-occurring substance use disorders, so while it is difficult to make a conclusive diagnosis of, for example, a generalized anxiety disorder in a patient with such significant substance use, further questioning could help illuminate to what extent anxiety symptoms predated any substance use. All of her medical, psychiatric, and substance use challenges are exacerbated by psychosocial stressors. She is estranged from her family and has no significant community support system. She has legal issues and has apparently struggled to sustain employment. She is undomiciled which is a significant cause of stress and anxiety for those experiencing it and a significant barrier to engagement in any kind of treatment. Due to her substance use pattern and psychosocial stressors, she is at an increased chronic safety risk; however, she is not an acute safety risk as she is not expressing any suicidal ideation nor does she have any known history of suicide attempts. Securing her agreement to contact collateral sources of information (although it appears unlikely from her description of her level of support) could be helpful in verifying the key data informing this assessment. A comprehensive treatment plan for Lilly should address the issues mentioned above in order to provide her with the best possibility for sustained abstinence from substances.

## Conclusion

When a patient presents for assessment of a substance-related disorder, it is a critical opportunity to intervene. Ineffective assessments of substance-related disorders frequently stem from too narrow a focus on substance use, neglecting the medical and psychiatric domains and failing to consider how these three areas may interact. Successful assessments of substance use consider these dimensions and incorporate the patient's readiness to change. Patients must navigate a multitude of barriers to care including psychosocial stressors, complex treatment systems, and fear of being disbelieved or stigmatized while in substance use treatment, all of which can make the substance use assessment particularly challenging. Ultimately, however, a thorough and compassionate assessment of the medical, psychiatric, and substance use domains could be the catalyst for a patient making the decision to change an unhealthy pattern of substance use [17, 18].

**Key Points**

- A comprehensive substance use assessment must include attention to the medical and psychiatric domains, either or both of which may be contributing to the current presentation in addition to any substance use.
- Gathering a substance use history must include attention to the basic facts about use—some of which may be urgently needed for lifesaving purposes—as well as the patient's subjective experience of their use and thoughts about change.
- Patients who use substances may be reluctant to discuss their use in depth, particularly at an initial encounter.

## References


1. Woody GE, Cacciola J. Diagnosis and classification of DSM-IV-TR and ICD-10. In: Ruiz P, Strain EC, editors. Lowinson and Ruiz's substance abuse: a comprehensive textbook. 5th ed. Philadelphia: Lippincott Williams & Wilkins; 2011. p. 117.
2. Langenbucher J. In: Martin S, Suhr JA, editors. The Cambridge handbook of clinical assessment and diagnosis (Cambridge handbooks in psychology, Chap 28). Cambridge: Cambridge University Press; 2020.
3. Cacciola JS, et al. Development and initial evaluation of the Brief Addiction Monitor (BAM). J Subst Abus Treat. 2013;44(3):256–63.
4. SAMHSA/CSAT Treatment Improvement Protocols (TIP). Rockville (MD): Substance Abuse and Mental Health Services Administration (US); 2009. Available from: https://www.ncbi.nlm.nih.gov/books/NBK82999/.
5. Alterman AI, et al. Measurement of mental health in substance use disorder outpatients. J Subst Abus Treat. 2010;39(4):408–14.
6. National Institute on Alcohol Abuse and Alcoholism: Helping Patients Who Drink Too Much: A Clinician's Guide. 2005 Edition. http://www.niaaa.nih.gov/guide.
7. Kendler KS, Davis CG, Kessler RC. The familial aggregation of common psychiatric and substance use disorders in the National Comorbidity Survey: a family history study. Br J Psychiatry. 1997;170:541–8.
8. Posner K, et al. The Columbia-suicide severity rating scale: initial validity and internal consistency findings from three multisite studies with adolescents and adults. Am J Psychiatr. 2011;168(12):1266–77.
9. Cottler LB, Robins LN, Helzer JE. The reliability of the CIDI-SAM: a comprehensive substance abuse interview. Br J Addict. 1989;84(7):801–14.
10. Parran TV, McCormick RA, Cacciola JS. Chapter 20. In: Ries RK, editor. Principles of addiction medicine. 4th ed. Lippincott Williams &Wilkins; 2009.
11. American Psychiatric Association. Diagnostic and Statistical Manual IV, t.e. Arlington: American Psychiatric Publishing; Arlington, VA. 2013.
12. Prochaska JO, DiClemente CC. In: Miller WR, Heather N, editors. Treating addictive behavior: process of change. Springer Science & Business Media; New York, NY. 2013.
13. Miller WR, Tonigan SJ. Assessing drinkers' motivation for change: the Stages of Change Readiness and Treatment Eagerness Scale (SOCRATES). Psychol Addict Behav. 1996;10:81.

14. Dube SR, et al. The impact of adverse childhood experiences on health problems: evidence from four birth cohorts dating back to 1900. Prev Med. 2003;37(3):268–77.
15. Basu D, et al. Initial treatment dropout in patients with substance use disorders attending a tertiary care de-addiction Centre in North India. Indian J Med Res. 2017;146(Supplement):S77–84.
16. Avery J, et al. Improvement in Residents' attitudes toward individuals with substance use disorders following an online training module on stigma. HSS J. 2019;15(1):31–6.
17. Gilburt H, Drummond C, Sinclair J. Navigating the alcohol treatment pathway: a qualitative study from the service users' perspective. Alcohol Alcohol. 2015;50(4):444–50.
18. Solberg H, Naden D. It is just that people treat you like a human being: the meaning of dignity for patients with substance use disorders. J Clin Nurs. 2020;29(3–4):480–91.

# Neurobiology of Substance Use Disorders

# 2

Manesh Gopaldas and Kristopher A. Kast

## Introduction

The past two decades of neuroscience research in preclinical and clinical models have significantly enhanced our understanding of the neurobiology of addiction. Koob and Volkow have summarized a large and growing body of literature, proposing a three-stage model of substance-related and addictive disorders [1]. Recently, Kwako and colleagues proposed that this three-stage model could provide a clinically applicable framework for diagnosis and treatment [2]. In this chapter, we present a clinical case, review the three-stage model, and apply this neuroscience-based framework to clinical care.

## Clinical Case

We begin with a case to illustrate some problems confronting the clinician caring for individuals with substance use and related disorders. This case calls attention to observational data that are helpfully organized and made clinically useful by a neuroscience-based framework.

M. Gopaldas
Department of Psychiatry and Behavioral Sciences, Vanderbilt University Medical Center, Nashville, TN, USA
e-mail: manesh.m.gopaldas@vumc.org

K. A. Kast (✉)
Department of Psychiatry and Behavioral Sciences, Vanderbilt University School of Medicine, Addiction Consult Service, Vanderbilt University Medical Center, Nashville, TN, USA
e-mail: kristopher.a.kast@vumc.org



J. D. Avery, D. Hankins (eds.), *Addiction Medicine*, Psychiatry Update 2,
https://doi.org/10.1007/978-3-030-86430-9_2

## History of Present Illness

You are asked to assess "Mr. M," a 35-year-old man with a history of unspecified anxiety and depressive disorders who presents to the emergency department in distress, requesting hospitalization to address worsening suicidal ideation. Your open-ended questions elicit prominent, unrelenting symptoms of anxiety and sleep-onset insomnia that are "only" relieved by alcohol use – though he ruminates aloud that his drinking "to get going" in the morning is now affecting his work and personal responsibilities.

You find that Mr. M's alcohol intake escalated over preceding months to five 12-ounce beers four times per week, with one or two "heavier" binges causing episodic amnesia. As if anticipating chastisement, he reports "And every time I try to stop, I can't sleep – I start shaking – and my body just starts to feel like it is shutting down… like I'm going to die."

## Psychosocial History

Mr. M's neurodevelopmental history is notable for significant childhood adversity, including emotional and physical abuse by an older brother, with subsequent impairing anxiety in nearly all social situations "for as long as [he] could remember." He worries about how others perceive him and engages in self-evaluative thoughts and post-event processing. His intense ruminations often result in hopelessness and anticipatory worry about future social interactions, though these symptoms have gone undiagnosed and untreated throughout his child- and early adulthood.

He recalls first trying alcohol in college, quickly learning that drinking alleviated many of his anxiety symptoms. He began to identify with an intoxicated self-state: "It let me be myself." Initially, Mr. M consumed alcohol only in social settings, but his use extended over time to drinking alone, especially when overwhelmed with ruminative generalized worries. He tells you, "I noticed that I didn't really enjoy drinking anymore… but when I started worrying, I would be drinking before I even realized what I was doing."

Mr. M took a leave of absence midway through his second collegiate semester due to his symptoms, and he did not return. He now lives alone with few relationships, continuing to work in sales despite job dissatisfaction.

## Inpatient Hospital Course

After reviewing your diagnostic assessment and treatment recommendations, Mr. M agrees to voluntary inpatient admission for acute stabilization. Given his heavy alcohol use, presenting blood alcohol level (<100 mg/dL), and history of moderate withdrawal symptoms, you begin a symptom-triggered protocol for alcohol withdrawal treatment. Moderate doses of diazepam provide acute withdrawal symptom relief and allow you to discuss further post-acute treatment options for his comorbid alcohol use and anxiety disorders. He chooses extended-release naltrexone with close outpatient follow-up in your addiction clinic, deferring other interventions: "I'm a lot less anxious after the [diazepam]."

## Outpatient Clinic Management

Two weeks post-discharge, Mr. M presents to your office. He arrives late and appears apprehensive, with psychomotor activation (fidgeting, frequent repositioning), avoidant eye contact, and brisk speech, at times fumbling over his words. He reports muscle tension, restlessness, sweating, and trouble concentrating since discharge, with associated racing thoughts, excessive worrying, and panic-like episodes in public settings – "like being here." Despite having "urges" to use alcohol, he has remained abstinent, citing his strong "willpower." With guided questions, you are also able to identify limited adaptive coping strategies he has utilized (e.g., exercise, reading).

You review his untreated anxiety symptoms, their relationship to relapse risk, and recommend additional pharmacological and behavioral treatments to facilitate his recovery.

## Discussion

In this section, we introduce the chronic disease model of addiction and review the three neurofunctional domains implicated in the development and maintenance of substance use and related disorders.

## Addiction Cycle

Addiction is a chronic, relapsing illness that involves distress or functional impairment due to intense desire for a drug, loss of control over its use, and profound discomfort with abstinence [3]. Individuals with substance-related and addictive disorders experience this maladaptive pattern of use repetitively and compulsively, often despite harmful consequences.

Koob and Volkow have characterized addiction as a recurring cycle of three distinct stages: (1) binge/intoxication, (2) withdrawal/negative affect, and (3) preoccupation/anticipation [1]. The binge/intoxication stage is marked by reward and positive reinforcement, where the drug serves to promote positive subjective experience [4]. The withdrawal/negative affect stage is an aversive, stress-like state marked by negative reinforcement, where drug consumption serves to remove the discomfort experienced during abstinence [4]. The preoccupation/anticipation stage is characterized by executive function deficits and impulsivity, which contribute to drug craving and increase risk of relapse.

## Neuroanatomy and Circuits

The neurocircuitry of each stage has been well characterized in rodent studies, with corroborating human subject evidence [1]. We review this overlapping neurocircuitry in detail below.

### Binge/Intoxication

All known substances associated with addictive syndromes affect the reward system – centered around a group of structures located in the basal ganglia [5]. Midbrain neurons projecting to the striatum (and the prefrontal cortex) release dopamine tonically and, to a lesser extent, opioid peptides [1]. These neurotransmitters are responsible for (1) positively valenced emotions (e.g., euphoria) with increased firing in the ventromedial striatum and (2) increased behaviors that seek anticipated reward via the dorsolateral striatum. These midbrain-originating circuits are termed (1) the mesolimbic dopamine pathway, which projects to the nucleus accumbens (NAcc) and mediates reward and reinforcement, and (2) the nigrostriatal dopamine pathway, which projects to the dorsolateral striatum, controlling habitual motor functions [5].

Repeated substance-induced dopamine release in the NAcc leads to anticipatory dopamine activity in the reward circuit when re-exposed to substance-related cues, producing *incentive salience* for these cues [1]. Repeated use further results in compensatory neuroadaptations that attenuate substance-induced dopamine release. A new, lowered set point for tonic dopaminergic activity is established (a process termed allostasis), with the downstream effect of diminished reward response to natural reinforcers. Ultimately, most patients presenting for treatment experience heightened cue-related incentive salience, less substance-induced euphoria, and low expectations of reward from non-substance activities (e.g., relationships, work).

### Withdrawal/Negative Affect

Two neurobiological mechanisms – within- and between-system neuroadaptations – are thought to underlie the experience of acute and post-acute withdrawal [6]. With chronic substance use, within-system changes counter rewarding effects by downregulating reward signaling in the NAcc via allostasis, producing a relative dopaminergic deficit. The between-system changes, in contrast, are characterized by enhanced recruitment of stress circuits in the extended amygdala – sometimes termed the "anti-reward" system. The extended amygdala consists of several structures including the central nucleus of the amygdala (CeA), bed nucleus of the stria terminalis (BNST), and shell of the NAcc.

This anti-reward system upregulation results in elevated levels of amygdalar corticotropin-releasing factor (CRF), norepinephrine (NE), and dynorphin, as well as activation of the hypothalamic-pituitary-adrenal (HPA) axis [7]. Acute and post-acute withdrawals are associated with relative upregulation of the HPA axis, resulting in increased adrenocorticotropic hormone, corticosterone, and amygdalar

CRF. These neuroadaptations collectively produce a stress-like state marked by negative affect (i.e., irritability, emotional pain, anxiety, and dysphoria) that is prolonged beyond the acute withdrawal state (lasting from weeks to years) and also drives negative reinforcement processes responsible for craving and relapse [4].

### Preoccupation/Anticipation

Impairments in decision-making, self-regulation, and behavioral inhibition are often observed in individuals with substance use disorders. These executive function deficits contribute significantly to relapsing behavior despite accumulating negative consequences.

To conceptualize cognitive control of impulsive and compulsive behavior, two heuristically useful and opposing prefrontal cortical circuits have been proposed: a "Go system" mediated by the anterior cingulate and dorsolateral prefrontal cortex and a "Stop system" mediated by the ventrolateral and orbitofrontal cortex [1]. When presented with the incentive salience of a substance-related cue (e.g., reward craving when passing a liquor store) or the aversive withdrawal state (e.g., relief craving when waking the morning after a binge), these two systems engage (Go system) or inhibit (Stop system) the associated habitual substance-seeking behavior. In the above examples, the Go system would initiate recurrent drinking, while the Stop system may prioritize an abstinence goal. A relatively upregulated Go system and downregulated Stop system result in a decisional balance tipped toward relapsing behaviors.

## Treatment

In this section, we interpret Mr. M's clinical case within the three-stage model and describe the utility of the Addictions Neuroclinical Assessment. Select pharmacological and behavioral treatments for substance use disorders are then reviewed within this neuroscience framework.

### Translating Neuroscience into Clinical Practice

Developed by the National Institute on Alcohol Abuse and Alcoholism (NIAAA), the Addictions Neuroclinical Assessment (ANA) provides the building blocks of the Alcohol and Addiction Research Domain Criteria (AARDoC) [8]. The ANA is a neuroscience-based assessment tool that incorporates the three-stage model of addiction. It includes behavioral, self-report, and neuroimaging measures for each stage, allowing for more precise diagnosis and treatment of addictive disorders.

Kwako and colleagues evaluated the ANA framework in a sample of patients with alcohol use disorders (AUDs), showing that the three-stage model corresponds to three clinically identifiable neurofunctional domains: incentive salience, negative emotionality, and executive (dys)function [2]. Furthermore, the study identified factors that either predicted development or indicated the presence of dysregulation within the three neurofunctional domains. These findings help us to better understand how AUD may develop and to begin to classify different subtypes of AUD.

Further, applying the three-stage neurobiological framework to a specific case provides a clinically useful heuristic for diagnostic assessment and treatment planning. For example, Mr. M reports significant cravings for alcohol prior to attending social events, illustrating an associative learning process involved in *incentive salience*: socially cued anxiety and alcohol use become a learned association, with resulting reinforced and intensified subjective experience of "wanting" alcohol when exposed to social cues. Mr. M's worsened anxiety and insomnia when attempting to reduce his drinking further demonstrate compensatory allostatic changes in stress-response systems corresponding with *negative emotionality*: abstinence states lead to acute and post-acute withdrawal symptoms elicited by within-system downregulation of normal dopaminergic functioning and between-system upregulation of the anti-reward circuitry. And finally, his relapsing alcohol use – despite his own concern for its sequelae – in response to relief cravings during anxious rumination shows a relative imbalance between his Go and Stop systems, expressing *executive (dys)function*.

In addition, Mr. M's case overlapped with several predictors and indicators of vulnerability in each neurofunctional domain as identified in the AUD cohort studied by Kwako and colleagues. His history of emotional abuse predicts risk across all three domains, perhaps mediated by epigenetic mechanisms [8]. Among the identified indicators of current dysfunction, Mr. M's elevated anxiety and depressive symptoms are associated with the incentive salience and negative emotionality domains, perhaps mediated by the maladaptive learning and anti-reward system upregulation described above.

Mr. M's treatment course may be understood as targeting each of these neurofunctional domains. As with most patients presenting for substance use treatment, his *withdrawal/negative emotionality* features prominently at the outset. Immediate attention is paid to stabilizing acute withdrawal symptoms via agonist therapy, a concept applicable to several substance categories (including nicotine, opioid, and alcohol, among others). Restoring relative GABA-ergic tone via benzodiazepine therapy reduces acute withdrawal symptoms (and mitigates risk of severe withdrawal, including seizure or delirium). Other acute withdrawal treatments target the upregulated stress-response/anti-reward system directly, as with lofexidine and clonidine targeting noradrenergic hyperactivity in opioid withdrawal.

Ameliorating the immediate aversive state allows for initial engagement in educational, motivational, and relapse-prevention interventions. No longer overwhelmed by relief cravings, an imbalanced Go/Stop cognitive control system may be engaged by psychosocial and psychotherapeutic interventions in a targeted way.

Education and cue avoidance feature prominently in early treatment. Identifying high-risk situations is an early goal in cognitive-behavioral treatment of substance use disorders, similar to the 12-step directive to change "people, places, and things" associated with prior use. Both interventions diminish the contribution of incentive salience to relapse risk and intend to allow this maladaptive learning to extinguish over time, while new associations form in the context of substance-abstaining activities and relationships.

However, avoidance of all cue-related incentive salience is rarely achievable, and often relapse prevention is further aided by pharmacotherapy that reduces reward- and relief-craving experiences. Effective maintenance agonist and antagonist therapies – such as nicotine, methadone, buprenorphine, and naltrexone – typically occupy a target receptor for the relevant substance, partly reducing the effect of dopaminergic firing with re-exposure to cues or recurrent substance use. For individuals with AUD, the mu-opioid receptor antagonist naltrexone reduces cravings and risk of relapse or heavy use – demonstrating a link between the opioidergic system and alcohol use in this population [9]. Overall, patients on these therapies report reduced cravings and cognitive preoccupation with substance-related themes, theoretically creating cognitive space for engagement in psychosocial interventions.

Diagnosis and treatment of co-occuring psychiatric disorders further address dysfunction within each neurofunctional domain. As in Mr. M's case, targeted medication and psychotherapeutic treatment of anxiety and depressive symptoms implicated in the negative emotionality domain may further mitigate risk of relapse and/or facilitate engagement in an ongoing treatment relationship. Behavioral activation and engagement with a recovery-supportive social network may further improve mood and anxiety symptoms while simultaneously reducing exposure to high-risk contexts (e.g., social isolation or use-associated environments and contacts). And cognitive behavioral interventions, like identification and reappraisal of cognitive distortions, engage cognitive control networks in adaptive learning that may mitigate imbalanced Go/Stop system decision-making (see Fig. 2.1).

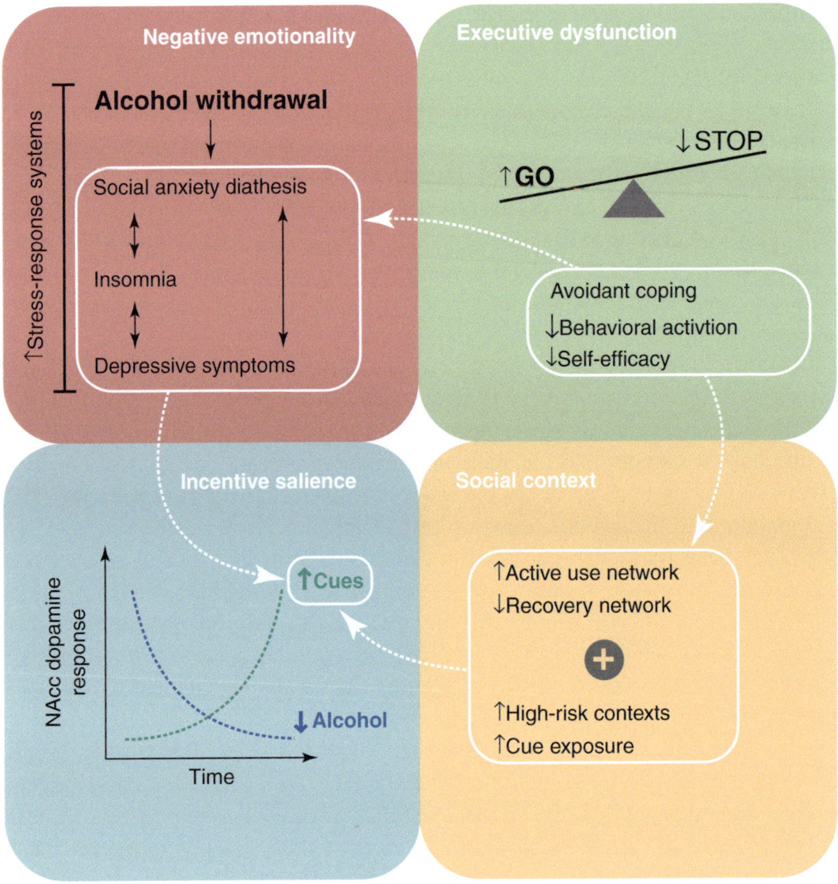


**Fig. 2.1** The interaction of three neurobiological domains with social context in Mr. M, an individual with alcohol use disorder. The three neurobiological domains include (1) negative emotionality, (2) executive dysfunction, and (3) incentive salience; each interacts with components of the other domains and surrounding social context to contribute to the risk of relapsing alcohol use. Within negative emotionality, an upregulated stress-response system occurs in the context of acute and post-acute alcohol withdrawal, which exacerbates Mr. M's insomnia and underlying social anxiety and depressive symptoms. Executive dysfunction, with imbalanced Go/Stop cognitive control, reinforces avoidant coping and reduces behavioral activation, decreasing Mr. M's self-efficacy and contributing to learned helplessness. Over time, allostatic changes in the reward system lead to reduced response to alcohol itself, with relatively heightened response to its associated cues; in Mr. M's case, incentive salience becomes associated with negative internal emotional states and high-risk social contexts, further increasing risk of relapse when exposed to these cues

## References

1. Koob GF, Volkow ND. Neurobiology of addiction: a neurocircuitry analysis. Lancet Psychiatry. 2016;3(8):760–73.
2. Kwako LE, Schwandt ML, Ramchandani VA, et al. Neurofunctional domains derived from deep behavioral phenotyping in alcohol use disorder. Am J Psychiatry. 2019;176(9):744–53.
3. McLellan AT, Lewis DC, O'Brien CP, et al. Drug dependence, a chronic medical illness: implications for treatment, insurance, and outcomes evaluation. JAMA. 2000;284:1689–95.
4. Koob GF, Mason BJ. Existing and future drugs for the treatment of the dark side of addiction. Annu Rev Pharmacol Toxicol. 2016;56(1):299–322.
5. Ries RK, et al. The ASAM principles of addiction medicine. Wolters Kluwer Health, Philadelphia, PA; 2014.
6. Koob GF. The dark side of emotion: the addiction perspective. Eur J Pharmacol. 2015;753:73–87.
7. Koob GF, Buck CL, Cohen A, et al. Addiction as a stress surfeit disorder. Neuropharmacology. 2014;76:370–82.
8. Kwako LE, Momenan R, Litten RZ, et al. Addictions neuroclinical assessment: a neuroscience-based framework for addictive disorders. Biol Psychiatry. 2016;80(3):179–89.
9. Hendershot CS, Wardell JD, Samokhvalov AV, et al. Effects of naltrexone on alcohol self-administration and craving: meta-analysis of human laboratory studies. Addict Biol. 2016;22:1515–27.

# Alcohol Use Disorder

# 3

Kseniya Svyatets

## Introduction

Alcohol use disorder is a highly prevalent illness, with tremendous morbidity, mortality, and strain on the healthcare system. In 2019, approximately 14 million adults and 400,000 adolescents met criteria for alcohol use disorder [1]. Recent data shows that alcoholism is the third leading cause of death in the United States [1, 2]. An estimated 261 deaths occur daily from alcohol use, with a loss of 29 years of life per death [3]. Alcohol abuse carries a significant socioeconomic burden as well. In 2010, alcohol misuse cost the United States $249.0 billion [1, 3], which included economic losses in workplace productivity, healthcare spending, law enforcement costs, and motor vehicle accidents [4]. An estimated two out of every five dollars spent on alcohol-related costs are covered by taxpayers [4]. There is no question that alcohol addiction directly and indirectly affects every member of our society.

With the pervasiveness of substance use disorders and their medical sequelae, addiction has become one of the most commonly encountered domains of illness in healthcare. A 2016 survey shows that approximately 80% of hospitalists and 35% of primary care providers reported routinely treating patients with addiction. This same survey showed that only 27% of hospitalists and 18% of primary care doctors felt fully confident in their ability to screen patients for substance use, 35% of hospitalists and 17% of primary care doctors considered themselves very prepared to diagnose addiction, and most notably only 12% of hospitalists and 9% of primary care physicians felt thoroughly prepared to engage patients in brief interventions [5]. Why do physicians feel such discomfort in treating this spectrum of illnesses? The same 2016 survey also showed that a large proportion of physicians believe that addiction is a choice, many find caring for patients with addiction less satisfying, and the majority of physicians consider disorders of addiction to be more

K. Svyatets (✉)
Addiction Psychiatry Fellow, New York University, New York, NY, USA
e-mail: Kseniya.Svyatets@nyulangone.org

 
J. D. Avery, D. Hankins (eds.), *Addiction Medicine*, Psychiatry Update 2,
https://doi.org/10.1007/978-3-030-86430-9_3

challenging to manage than other illnesses [5]. Substance use disorders remain highly stigmatized in our society, and healthcare personnel are not immune to these biases. These attitudes contribute to the numerous barriers to care that patients with addiction experience.

Psychiatrists are often consulted on patients struggling with alcohol use disorder. Common reasons for such consults include the high rate of comorbidities with primary psychiatric illness and discomfort of primary care/internal medicine doctors in working with this population. This chapter highlights the clinical case of a middle-aged man with severe alcohol use disorder and comorbid psychiatric pathology. This case serves to illustrate the numerous biopsychosocial factors at play in alcohol use disorder, the complexity of dual diagnosis, and the treatment options available for alcohol dependence.

## Case

Mr. B is a 42-year-old male, recently separated from his wife and children, employed in finance, with no prior psychiatric history, who was brought in to the emergency department by his brother for abdominal pain, intractable vomiting, lethargy, and dizziness. He was found to have alcoholic ketoacidosis and admitted to the medical unit for rehydration and electrolyte repletion. This was Mr. B's second admission for alcoholic ketoacidosis and fifth time in the hospital for alcohol-related complications. The other three were emergency room visits for trauma due to falls while intoxicated. Despite multiple hospital visits, Mr. B had never received counseling from his medical providers or referrals for addiction treatment. On his most recent admission, the hospitalist noted Mr. B's nonchalant attitude about his numerous hospitalizations and requested a psychiatric assessment.

Throughout the evaluation, Mr. B minimized his alcohol use and showed a limited understanding of the toll his addiction had taken on his life. He said that he came from a family of "casual drinkers." His parents would routinely have multiple glasses of wine with dinner and were often intoxicated after work. Mr. B recalled a childhood of frequent outbursts at home and occasional physical violence between his parents. His father had a lucrative job in finance and his mother was a manager in a prominent public relations firm. There was never any acknowledgment that his parents might have an unhealthy dependence on alcohol and potentially underlying mental health struggles. Mr. B's brother had several admissions to rehabs and continues in outpatient treatment for addiction, and he was characterized as the "black sheep" of the family.

Mr. B recalled that he had always been an anxious and "moody" person. As a teenager, he constantly worried over his future, whether he would get into a good college and live up to his parents' expectations. He would often find himself unable to relax and lose sleep over his worries. At times, he would be unable to eat due to his stress. He began having panic attacks in his senior year of high school. During these attacks, he would feel as if the walls were closing in on him; he could not breathe or focus. He says he has felt sad and empty for most of his life. There were multiple episodes throughout his life, during which he "fell into a dark hole." In those times, he would isolate himself in his room, avoid school and work, and spend days lying in bed. He occasionally had thoughts of not wanting to live anymore, but never formulated a plan to harm himself. These mood symptoms continued into adulthood, yet Mr. B never thought to seek mental health treatment. He believed that most people struggled with similar thoughts, and it was a matter of willpower to overcome them.

Mr. B began drinking with friends at age 15. His drinking was primarily social at first, but he soon realized that alcohol had a blunting effect on his anxiety and sadness. As he began his own career in finance, Mr. B's alcohol use increased exponentially. His career demanded perfectionism, long hours, and a competitive attitude. Alcohol helped him cope with his fear of failure and self-doubt. As Mr. B's drinking increased, he became more irritable with his family members, frequently intoxicated at family functions, and would occasionally sleep through events such as his children's sporting games. Mr. B reported experiencing tremulousness and anxiety when he attempted to cut back on his alcohol use. He denied a history of seizures, delirium tremens, or other episodes of complicated withdrawal. His wife expressed concerns many times over his increasing alcohol use, and several months ago, she separated from him. The week prior to his hospitalization, Mr. B had been drinking nearly a 750 mL bottle of whiskey daily.

Mr. B was reticent to discuss the notion that he may have a severe substance use disorder. He understood that his drinking had escalated into unhealthy patterns, yet he believed that alcohol played a significant role in helping him manage his stress. He expressed a goal of decreasing his alcohol intake but was not interested in complete alcohol cessation. The consulting psychiatrist provided psychoeducation on the nature of alcohol addiction and introduced treatment options including inpatient rehab, outpatient referrals, and medication-assisted treatment for alcohol use. Mr. B was strongly urged to consider inpatient rehab; however, he did not feel his alcohol use was severe enough to warrant inpatient care or medications. Mr. B did accept the psychiatrist's assessment that he likely meets criteria for generalized anxiety disorder and recurrent major depression, and he accepted a referral for an outpatient dual diagnosis clinic.

## Discussion

Mr. B's case illustrates how addiction develops gradually over time and negatively affects numerous aspects of a person's life. An awareness of the biopsychosocial factors at play can help build rapport, empathy, and understanding of the patient, as well as aid in the prompt diagnosis and treatment of patients, including those who may feel uncomfortable disclosing the full extent of their substance use. Mr. B's history includes several determinants which increased his risk for substance abuse. From a biological perspective, Mr. B has significant genetic loading toward alcohol use. His brother struggled with a severe alcohol use disorder, and both parents had substantial alcohol misuse, the full extent of which is unclear. Some literature estimates that genetics are 60% responsible for the formation of alcoholism, while the other 40% is determined by psychological and social factors. Other biological theories postulate that family history of alcoholism increases the risk of a patient developing alcohol use disorder by three to four times [6]. Mr. B also reports long-standing untreated symptoms of anxiety and depression. Mood disorders are a well-documented risk factor for developing substance use disorders. An estimated 30–40% of people with alcohol addiction have comorbid depression, 25–50% meet criteria for an anxiety disorder, and approximately 10–15% have a history of suicidality [6].

There are multiple psychological theories about personality structures which predispose to addiction. Classic psychoanalysis postulates that patients with alcohol addiction are fixed in the oral stage of development [6]. Kohut and Balint theorized that patients with addiction utilize alcohol as a means to replace missing self-esteem and inner peace [7]. Other psychodynamic theories claim that addiction to substances may be an attempt to control unacceptable affective states including anger, guilt, shame, and sadness [7]. An initial psychiatric consultation is insufficient for appreciating the full psychodynamic influences at play. However, from Mr. B's history, it is reasonable to hypothesize that self-esteem and painful emotional states may have been another predisposing factor for him to addiction. Lastly, societal attitudes strongly affect a patient's propensity toward alcohol use. Mr. B grew up in an environment where his parents frequently drank to the point of intoxication. He continued in a career where colleagues were frequently socializing with one another outside of work and using alcohol and drugs while doing so. He was constantly exposed to a social normalization of severe alcohol use, and these experiences likely hindered his realization of how problematic his own alcohol use had become.

An integral aspect of any psychiatric evaluation in a patient with suspected alcohol use disorder is assessment for comorbid psychiatric pathology. Chronic substance use can induce numerous mood states including depression, anxiety, neurovegetative symptoms, mania, and psychosis. Alcohol intoxication is specifically known to precipitate mood lability, while alcohol withdrawal exacerbates anxiety and insomnia [8]. Differentiating between alcohol-induced mood states and primary psychiatric disorders is often a challenge for even the seasoned psychiatrist. In order to make the distinction, it is important to obtain a timeline of the onset of mood symptoms and substance use. If the patient has had significant periods of sobriety during which he experienced mood symptoms, he would likely meet criteria for a primary psychiatric disorder such as major depressive disorder. Another clue is that substance-induced mood symptoms will resolve or at least significantly decrease in the first few weeks of abstinence while primary psychiatric symptoms will persist. For this reason, some psychiatrists choose to defer treatment for primary mood states, barring any acute need, until after a few weeks of sobriety are achieved. Mr. B reports a clear childhood history of anxiety and depression, which began prior to his onset of alcohol use. He also notes that he used alcohol to help him manage these symptoms. In his case, he would meet criteria for a primary anxiety and depressive disorder, and initiation of an SSRI would have been reasonable, had he been amenable.

## Treatment

### Medical Complications

Treatment of alcohol use disorder is multifaceted and includes assessment for acute medical complications, evaluation for psychiatric comorbidities, and discussion of medication-assisted and psychosocial treatment options. The following discussion lists several medical complications which providers commonly encounter when consulting on patients with alcohol abuse. The full list of medical complications of chronic alcohol use is vast and beyond the scope of this chapter.

The first step in providing treatment for a patient struggling with chronic alcohol abuse is to effectively manage withdrawal. Symptoms to monitor include nausea, vomiting, increased anxiety, tremors, sensory disturbances, and disorientation. The Clinical Institute Withdrawal Assessment for Alcohol (CIWA) scale is the measure of alcohol withdrawal most commonly used by healthcare professionals and incorporates both objective and subjective data on the above domains of withdrawal symptoms. Long-acting benzodiazepines are the treatment of choice for withdrawal; however in patients with liver compromise, it is safer to use benzodiazepines that do not undergo hepatic conjugation such as lorazepam and oxazepam [2].

Inadequate treatment of alcohol withdrawal can lead to serious medical complications including seizures and delirium tremens. Seizures occur in about 1% of patients who are untreated for withdrawal, and patients are at highest risk in the first three days of withdrawal [2]. Delirium tremens (DTs) is a rare phenomenon marked by autonomic instability, delirium, and hallucinations. Approximately 5% of patients in alcohol withdrawal develop DTs, and the risk is again highest within the first three days of withdrawal [2]. Previously, DTs had a mortality rate of about 30%; however with medical advances, the mortality rate has decreased to 1% [9]. Both DTs and seizures are treated with high-dose rapid-onset IV benzodiazepines. ICU management is often required for patients in DTs as they require constant monitoring and can deteriorate rapidly. Patients in withdrawal refractory to benzodiazepines are often administered phenobarbital [2]. Antiepileptic medications are sometimes used prophylactically to prevent seizures; however data is limited.

Some patients may ultimately be referred for inpatient detoxification ("detox") treatment. The patients referred for inpatient detoxification are typically those who have expressed an interest in stopping alcohol after chronic use and for whom there is some concern—either through high volume of use or due to past complicated alcohol withdrawal—that the early phase of alcohol cessation could result in complicated withdrawal. Inpatient detoxification typically lasts no more than one week and incorporates medical treatment for withdrawal symptoms and various psychosocial and psychotherapeutic substance abuse treatment modalities. Treatment with inpatient detoxification is generally not an effective long-term treatment for alcohol use disorder; over half of those who participate are using alcohol again within two weeks of discharge, with over 80% ultimately drinking again [15].

Alcohol hallucinosis is a syndrome sometimes mistaken for DTs. Patients with alcohol hallucinosis experience visual hallucinations without delirium or autonomic instability, although other kinds of hallucinations have been reported as well. Alcohol hallucinosis is usually time limited; although most situations will eventually resolve without pharmacological management, short-term antipsychotics are often helpful for the comfort of the patient [2].

Wernicke-Korsakoff syndrome is another set of medical complications that psychiatrists may encounter in chronic alcohol users. Wernicke-Korsakoff is in reality two distinct syndromes caused by thiamine deficiency, as a result of decreased oral intake in the context of chronic alcohol abuse. Wernicke's disease is characterized by symptoms of ocular dysfunction, gait disturbances, and mental status changes. Most patients do not present with all three symptoms; therefore, Wernicke's should be suspected in all alcoholic patients who present with an acute development of any of these symptoms. Wernicke's is a medical emergency, as lack of prompt treatment can lead to Korsakoff syndrome or death in a significant number of patients. Korsakoff syndrome is a chronic memory disorder, marked by retrograde and anterograde amnesia, which occurs as a result of long-standing thiamine deficiency. Wernicke's is treated with high-dose intravenous thiamine, as oral thiamine is not absorbed well, and multivitamins [2]. Korsakoff syndrome is considered irreversible and there is limited data on treatment options; however, high-dose thiamine is typically used.

## Medication-Assisted Treatment

Patients with moderate to severe alcohol use disorder would benefit from a conversation about medication-assisted treatment options. Currently, the three medications approved by the US Food and Drug Administration (FDA) for alcohol use disorder are naltrexone, disulfiram, and acamprosate. Naltrexone is an opioid receptor antagonist and is also FDA approved for opiate addiction. By blocking the opioid receptors, naltrexone is believed to reduce the dopamine-enhancing effects of alcohol, thereby reducing cravings and feelings of intoxication [10]. Patients who initiate naltrexone must not have taken opiates for 7–10 days prior; otherwise, the opioid blockade of naltrexone will precipitate withdrawal. Naltrexone is often a first-line choice for patients due to the easy once a day dosing. Naltrexone also comes in a monthly depot formation, improving efficacy in patients who have difficulty taking pills daily. Notable side effects of naltrexone include nausea, abdominal pain, vomiting, CNS disturbances, hepatotoxicity, and rarely suicidal ideation. Due to the risk of hepatotoxicity, routine monitoring of liver function tests is highly recommended. Acamprosate is an alternative medication to naltrexone, often used when patients are unable to tolerate the side effects of naltrexone or have liver compromise, since it is renally cleared. The mechanism of acamprosate is not fully understood; however it is believed to counter the hyperglutamatergic state that emerges in the brain after repeated cycles of alcohol intoxication and withdrawal. Acamprosate has few side effects and few drug interactions [10]. It is not known to cause hepatotoxicity and is a good option for patients with significant liver dysfunction, although it cannot be used in patients with renal impairment. One downside to acamprosate is the requirement for three times daily dosing, which can be challenging for some patients to manage. Disulfiram is the third and oldest FDA-approved medication for alcohol use disorder. Disulfiram blocks aldehyde dehydrogenase, creating a buildup of toxic acetaldehyde when patients consume alcohol. When a patient drinks while taking disulfiram, they experience a highly unpleasant reaction to the acetaldehyde which may include nausea, vomiting, sweating, flushing, blood pressure fluctuations, palpitations, and rarely cardiac issues [10]. Evidence for the efficacy of disulfiram for alcohol cessation is inconsistent; however, it is a good option for highly motivated patients for whom the prospect of the disulfiram reaction is an effective deterrent to alcohol use.

FDA-approved medications for alcohol use disorder

| Medication name | FDA year of approval | Dosing | Common side effects |
|---|---|---|---|
| Disulfiram | 1951 | Once daily | Nausea, vomiting, sweating, flushing, blood pressure fluctuations, palpitations, and rarely cardiac issues when ingested with alcohol |
| Naltrexone | 1984 | Once daily or monthly IM depot | Nausea, abdominal pain, vomiting, CNS disturbances, hepatotoxicity, and rarely suicidal ideation |
| Acamprosate | 2004 | TID dosing | Few side effects, most commonly diarrhea |

Gabapentin, topiramate, and valproic acid are not approved by the FDA but are common second-line agents for alcohol use disorder. Gabapentin is particularly helpful for patients with alcohol use disorder and comorbid anxiety or neuropathic pain. Topiramate has some data for efficacy in both alcohol use disorder and cocaine use disorder and is sometimes used for patients who struggle with comorbid substance abuse. Valproic acid is an appropriate choice to consider in patients with bipolar disorder or severe mood lability and alcohol use disorder. It is best to utilize FDA-approved treatment options as the first-line management for alcohol use disorder; however, these agents can be helpful adjuncts to consider.

## Inpatient Treatments

As discussed earlier, inpatient detoxification may be considered for some patients where there is concern for medically complicated acute alcohol withdrawal and who want additional support and treatment in the early phase of cessation. Longer-term treatments, often colloquially referred to as "rehab," may last from weeks to months and typically offer intensive treatment in a variety of modalities (including psychotherapy and medication-assisted treatment) to support abstinence from alcohol. Patients will often need to be medically cleared for admission to these rehabilitation facilities out of concern for their ability to manage severe alcohol withdrawal, either by completing a brief detoxification first or by confirmation that the patient has not experienced complicated alcohol withdrawal in the past when stopping. Important considerations for helping a patient select one of these longer-term rehabilitation facilities include treatment modalities offered, length of the program, insurance coverage, and cost. Finally, some patients who have severe alcohol use disorder and a decompensated co-occurring mental health diagnosis (such as major depression, bipolar disorder, or a psychotic illness) should be considered for admission to a dual-diagnosis psychiatric unit that can treat both alcohol and other substance use disorders as well as the co-occurring psychiatric disorder. These units are becoming less common, however, as the overall number of inpatient psychiatric beds is gradually being reduced.

## Psychosocial Interventions

Mr. B had been admitted five times for alcohol-related complications, yet the consulting psychiatrist was the first physician to provide counseling for addiction. This is not an uncommon scenario for patients. In contrast to other chronic medical conditions, such as diabetes, hypertension, and cancer, physicians feel uncomfortable and ill-prepared to provide counseling on addiction and too often avoid the topic altogether. Yet, evidence has shown that even brief time-limited interventions can have a significant impact on a patient's motivation to change. A Cochrane review from 2019 examined data from 69 studies and found that brief interventions by primary care physicians can reduce the average weekly amount of alcohol consumed in patients followed for up to a year after [11]. Brief interventions for alcohol use are varied and can encompass assessment of motivation for change, feedback about current use, and psychoeducation about pharmacological and behavioral options for behavioral modification [11]. One example of a straightforward brief intervention which can be done in any time-limited setting is known as the 5A framework: *Ask* about the use, *advise* to quit, *assess* desire to change, *assist* in quitting with medication and therapy, and *arrange* follow-up.

Motivational interviewing (MI) is known as the quintessential interviewing technique for patients struggling with ambivalence about alcohol and/or other substance use. MI aims to elicit patients' motivations for change through four core components: engaging the patient in conversation, focusing on an agenda, evoking patients' motivations for change, and planning for change if the patient is ready and agreeable. MI utilizes the core skills of open-ended questions, affirming patients' strengths and beliefs, reflective listening, and summarizing [12]. MI is a collaborative, non-confrontational style of interviewing and can be successfully utilized both in brief interventions and longer-standing therapeutic relationships.

For longer-term treatment, there is an ever-growing number of psychotherapeutic modalities that have been shown to be effective with addiction disorders. Cognitive behavioral therapy (CBT) is one of the most commonly used psychotherapy techniques, applicable to a wide range of mental illnesses. In CBT, therapists and clients collaboratively examine connections between thoughts, behaviors, and emotions. The cognitive component of CBT for alcohol use focuses on identifying and reframing cognitive distortions surrounding substance use, tracking the circumstances present at the time of cravings to drink, managing painful emotions that may lead to alcohol use, and exploring the significance of dysfunctional beliefs about alcohol and their relationship to patients' core beliefs about themselves. Behavioral techniques center around avoiding and managing triggers, tolerating cravings, and building healthy coping skills and new rituals without alcohol. Network Therapy, created by Dr. Marc Galanter in the 1990s, is a modality which brings the patients' loved ones into sessions, utilizing social support and community reinforcement as powerful motivational tools in the mutual goal of sobriety [13]. Acceptance and Commitment Therapy has gained traction in recent years, as a therapeutic technique that clarifies clients' values for committed action and utilizes mindfulness and cognitive defusion to manage triggers for alcohol use and painful emotions.

Group therapies are also powerful tools for patients with alcohol use disorder, providing clients with social support, peer mentorship, and reduction of stigma. Alcoholics Anonymous (AA) is one of the oldest and most well-known forms of group therapy, widely utilized in all states and many countries. A 2020 meta-analysis showed that AA performs at least as well if not better than other psychotherapeutic treatment options and may be particularly cost-effective compared to other treatments [14]. AA meetings focus on the 12 steps to recovery, which include admitting to powerlessness over alcohol, asking a higher power for forgiveness, and taking personal inventory of shortcomings. AA meetings also facilitate connections among individuals with alcohol use disorder at different points in their recovery; this kind of mutual support and use of personal experience can be particularly helpful for patients newly provided with a diagnosis of alcohol use disorder and questioning whether a life without regular alcohol use is possible. Different AA groups take different approaches to helping participants navigate the 12 steps, so if a patient with alcohol use disorder mentions a dislike for AA based on prior experience, it can be helpful to inquire about the specific issue that person had with AA and to mention that other AA groups might be a more positive experience for the patient. SMART Recovery groups are another group treatment option for patients. SMART Recovery uses a more cognitive-behavioral framework and may be particularly appealing for those patients who want a group treatment but have negative views on AA's focus on connecting with a higher power as part of treatment. Both AA and SMART Recovery are widely available and have options for in-person and virtual meetings.

It often takes numerous attempts at intervention before a patient moves forward from the precontemplative stage of addiction. In Mr. B's case, while the initial intervention by the psychiatrist did not result in an acceptance of treatment (a very common initial response to a medical provider's expression of concern about alcohol use), we can hope that it planted seeds of understanding of the nature of his addiction to alcohol and may result in more willingness to seek treatment in the future.

## Conclusion

Alcohol use disorder is a complex and varied illness which requires an interdisciplinary approach. Effective treatment combines medication-assisted treatment, psychosocial interventions, and management of comorbidities. Alcohol use disorder is a difficult illness to manage; however, given the vast associated morbidity and mortality, it is vital that the medical community continue to assess and treat it wherever possible in order to improve patient outcomes.

### Key Points

- Alcohol use disorder is one of the costliest illnesses in the United States and around the world both in terms of lives lost and its economic consequences.
- Every opportunity should be taken to screen and potentially intervene for patients for whom alcohol use disorder is suspected.
- Effective treatments for alcohol use disorder include three FDA-approved medications (disulfiram, acamprosate, and naltrexone) as well as other medication options that may help target co-occurring symptoms in addition to alcohol use disorder.
- Psychosocial treatments, including individual psychotherapy and groups, are effective for many people with alcohol use disorder and should be offered as an option along with medication-assisted treatments.

## References

1. National Institute on Alcohol Abuse and Alcoholism. [internet] NIH, Alcohol Facts and Statistics; 2020 Oct 30 [cited 2021 Jan 6]. Available from: https://www.niaaa.nih.gov/publications/brochures-and-fact-sheets/alcohol-facts-and-statistics.
2. Nisavic M, Nejad S. Patients with alcohol use disorder. In: Stern TA, Freudenreich O, Smith FA, Fricchione GL, Rosenbaum JF, editors. Massachusetts General Hospital handbook of general hospital psychiatry. Philadelphia: Saunders/Elsevier; 2018. p. 141–8.
3. Esser MB, Sherk A, Liu Y, Naimi TS, Stockwell T, Stahre M, et al. Deaths and years of potential life lost from excessive alcohol use – United States, 2011–2015. MMWR Morb Mortal Wkly Rep. 2020;69(30):981–7.
4. Alcohol and Public Health. [internet] Center for Disease Control and Prevention, Excessive Drinking is Draining the U.S. Economy; 2019, Dec 30 [cited 2021, Jan 6]. Available from: https://www.cdc.gov/alcohol/features/excessive-drinking.html.
5. Wakeman SE, Pham-Kanter G, Donelan K. Attitudes, practices, and preparedness to care for patients with substance use disorder: results from a survey of general internists. Subst Abus. 2016;37(4):635–41.
6. Sadock BJ, Sadock VA, Ruiz P. Alcohol-related disorders. In: Kaplan & Sadock's synopsis of psychiatry: Behavioral sciences/clinical psychiatry. 11th ed. Philadelphia: Wolters Kluwer; 2015. p. 624–39.
7. Gabbard GO. Substance-related and addictive disorders and eating disorders. In: Psychodynamic psychiatry in clinical practice. Washington, DC: American Psychiatric Press; 2014. p. 345–81.

8. Nunes EV, Weiss RD. Co-occurring mood and substance use disorders. In: Miller S, Fiellin DA, Rosenthal RN, Saitz R, American Society of Addiction Medicine, issuing body, editors. The ASAM principles of addiction medicine. Philadelphia: Lippincott Williams & Wilkins; 2019. p. 1360–88.
9. Wartenberg AA. Management of Alcohol Intoxication and Withdrawal. In: Miller S, Fiellin DA, Rosenthal RN, Saitz R, American Society of Addiction Medicine, issuing body, editors. The ASAM principles of addiction medicine. Philadelphia: Lippincott Williams & Wilkins; 2019. p. 1360–88. p. 704–22.
10. Kranzler HR, Soyka M. Diagnosis and pharmacotherapy of alcohol use disorder: a review. JAMA. 2018;320(8):815–24.
11. Beyer FR, Campbell F, Bertholet N, Daeppen JB, Saunders JB, Pienaar ED, Muirhead CR, Kaner EFS. The cochrane 2018 review on brief interventions in primary care for hazardous and harmful alcohol consumption: a distillation for clinicians and policy makers. Alcohol Alcohol. 2019;54(4):417–27.
12. Miller WR, Rollnick S. Motivational interviewing: helping people change. 3rd ed. New York: Guilford Press; 2013.
13. Galanter M, Dermatis H. Network therapy. In: Miller S, Fiellin DA, Rosenthal RN, Saitz R, American Society of Addiction Medicine, issuing body, editors. The ASAM principles of addiction medicine. Philadelphia: Lippincott Williams & Wilkins; 2019. p. 1360–88.
14. Kelly JF, Humphreys K, Ferri M. Alcoholics anonymous and other 12-step programs for alcohol use disorder. Cochrane Database Syst Rev. 2020;3:CD012880.
15. Manning V, Garfield JB, Staiger PK, Lubman DI, Lum JA, Reynolds J, Hall K, Bonomo Y, Lloyd-Jones M, Wiers RW, Piercy H. Effect of cognitive bias modification on early relapse among adults undergoing inpatient alcohol withdrawal treatment: a randomized clinical trial. JAMA Psychiat. 2021;78(2):133–40.

# Cannabis Use Disorder

# 4

Dhruti Patel

## Introduction

Cannabis continues to be the most widely used illicit substance in the United States. During the past decade, cannabis use disorders have increased in all age groups and sociodemographic groups [17]. This is partially reflective of a major shift in attitudes that is occurring in the United States and around the world both at the individual and at the broader policy level. In 1988, 24% of Americans supported legalization of cannabis; three decades later in 2018 that figure was 66% supporting legalization [10]. Although still illegal at the federal level, as of 2020 cannabis was legal in 11 US states plus the District of Columbia, with medical marijuana legal in dozens more states. Several states where legislative efforts have stopped short of full legalization have pursued a policy of decriminalization, eliminating penalties for possession of small amounts of cannabis for personal use.

Cannabis is available in multiple forms with varying concentrations of chemical compounds known as cannabinoids. Cannabinoids exert their effects through the endocannabinoid system by binding to cannabinoid receptors CB1 and CB2. The highest density of CB1 receptors is found in part of the brain that influences memory, concentration, pleasure, coordinated movements, and sensory and time perception [13]. The main cannabinoids are delta-9-tetrahydrocannabinol (THC) and cannabidiol (CBD). CBD, which is non-intoxicating, is FDA approved to treat two rare forms of childhood epilepsy. Its popularity has exploded in recent years as a largely unregulated treatment for a variety of ailments, particularly anxiety and several forms of chronic pain. The evidence to support its use for these other indications is mostly inconclusive, and patients interested in hearing more about CBD should be counseled on the lack of consistency among various preparations and the difficulty of knowing what these products actually contain. THC is the psychotropic

D. Patel (✉)
University of Miami Miller School of Medicine, Miami, FL, USA
e-mail: dhruti.patel@jhsmiami.org



J. D. Avery, D. Hankins (eds.), *Addiction Medicine*, Psychiatry Update 2,
https://doi.org/10.1007/978-3-030-86430-9_4

substance in cannabis primarily responsible for its intoxicating and psychogenic effects. THC activates the brain's reward system to release dopamine, and this flood of dopamine contributes to the pleasurable "high" that those who use seek. Long-term use, however, is associated with blunting of the dopamine system [3].

Acute cannabis intoxication for many people includes euphoria and sense of relaxation. However, potential adverse effects include anxiety, fear, paranoia, and acute psychosis with hallucinations and delusions. These effects are temporary in most cases, but appear to play a role in a subset of individuals in either precipitating or exacerbating chronic psychotic disorders. The risk of adverse effects increases with frequent use and with exposure to high concentrations of THC. The cannabis available today is much more potent than what was available in the past, with a THC to CBD ratio that has grown quickly in recent decades. One study of samples seized by the DEA between 1995 and 2014 showed an increase in potency from 4% to 12% and a THC to CBD ratio that increased from 14 to 80 over those two decades [8]. It is important to inquire about the method of use as concentrated products, commonly known as dabs or waxes, typically contain higher doses of THC and are more likely to produce adverse psychological symptoms. Use of edible cannabis can increase the risk of unintentional overdose due to its longer absorption time and delayed effect, often prompting the user to take a second dose. In addition, chronic users of cannabis are at risk for developing a condition known as cannabinoid hyperemesis syndrome (CHS), which is marked by severe cycles of nausea and vomiting which can lead individuals to make frequent trips to the emergency room. Supportive therapy is the mainstay of treatment for the syndrome, with patients reporting benefits from taking hot showers. It is shown to resolve when a person stops using cannabis [9].

While many people can use cannabis use without harm, a cannabis use disorder develops in approximately 9% of regular cannabis users [19, 20]. The DSM-5 defines cannabis dependence as a disorder characterized by continued problematic pattern of use leading to negative consequences that cause significant impairment or distress. For the full criteria based on the *Diagnostic and Statistical Manual of Mental Disorders – Fifth Edition* (DSM-5) criteria, see Table 4.1.

**Table 4.1** DSM criteria for cannabis use disorder

| |
|---|
| Using cannabis in larger amounts or over a longer period than was prescribed or intended |
| Making unsuccessful efforts to cut down or control cannabis use |
| Spending a lot of time in activities necessary to obtain, use, or recover from cannabis effects |
| Craving cannabis or feeling an urge to use cannabis |
| Failing to fulfill major life obligations at work, school, or home |
| Continuing to use cannabis despite persistent or recurrent social or interpersonal problems |
| Giving up or reducing involvement in important social, occupational, or recreational activities |
| Using cannabis in physically hazardous circumstances |
| Continuing to use cannabis despite having a persistent or recurrent physical or psychological problem |
| Tolerance, as defined by a need for markedly increased amounts of cannabis or a markedly diminished effect with continued use of the same amount of cannabis |
| Withdrawal, as manifested by the characteristic withdrawal syndrome |

Mild: 2–3 symptoms; moderate: 4–5 symptoms; severe: >6 symptoms

Cannabis use places individuals at risk for various adverse health consequences and may be associated with cognitive impairment, poor school or work performance, and psychiatric comorbidity such as mood disorders and psychosis. Common consequences include relationship and family problems, guilt associated with use of the drug, financial difficulties, low energy and self-esteem, dissatisfaction with productivity levels, sleep and memory problems, and low life satisfaction [7]. Most who use cannabis to the extent that they can be diagnosed with a use disorder perceive themselves as unable to stop, and most experience a withdrawal syndrome upon cessation.

Cannabis withdrawal is defined in the DSM-5 as clinically significant distress or impairment of social or occupational functioning seen approximately one week after cessation of heavy and prolonged use. Individuals typically experience irritability, anger, depression, sleep difficulty, craving, and decreased appetite. Onset of symptoms typically appears about 24 to 48 hours after the last cannabis use, peaks within four to six days, and lasts from one to three weeks, although significant individual differences occur in withdrawal expression [4]. The negative reinforcing effect of withdrawal makes relapse common in this period. Many indicate that these symptoms adversely impact their attempts to quit and motivate use of cannabis [6].

## Clinical Case

Anne is a 21-year-old college student, who was referred to the mental health clinic by her primary care physician for reporting changes in her mood. She says her mood is "okay" but reports having a high level of anxiety and has recently had a few episodes of overwhelming anxiety, shortness of breath, and chest pain.

As part of your assessment you inquire about her cannabis use. She tells you she smokes cannabis "socially." Upon further questioning she reveals that she smokes about one joint per day during the week and two or more joints per day on the weekend. She does not smoke tobacco and drinks "a few beers" weekly when at parties. She does not use any other substances. She first used cannabis in high school and initially only smoked in social settings. Over time, she has needed more cannabis to "take the edge off" and has strong cravings to use daily. She reports liking how cannabis decreases his anxiety and helps her fall asleep, although she thinks the cannabis sometimes makes her "paranoid," which results in her keeping away from friends and family at times. Furthermore, she explains she is failing two of her classes this year but was an excellent student in the past.

Anne has met the criteria for cannabis use disorder, and it is evident that her cannabis use is problematic and is likely causing or contributing to some of her school difficulties and medical conditions. After summarizing Anne's symptoms and counseling her on cannabis use disorder, Anne expresses that she was not aware of the addictive qualities of cannabis.

## Discussion

The public's increasing openness toward cannabis use has contributed to an increase in the number of cannabis users, which means more people who need treatment and intervention. Although more people are seeking help for problems with cannabis today, most who need treatment do not feel their use is problematic and are typically referred to treatment by others. There are also barriers to accessing help which commonly include fear of judgment, lack of knowledge of treatment options, long wait times for help, and lack of perceived need for help. Addressing a patient's cannabis use is often an ongoing process, requiring comprehensive assessment before a diagnosis can be made and in most cases frequent revisiting of the topic to assess shifts in the patient's attitude toward use.

## Screening

Medical providers for patients who struggle with cannabis use must become able to identify and characterize cannabis use disorders, provide education, and offer evidence-based treatments. The most basic facts to be obtained include amount used and frequency, duration of use, and route of administration. Taking a nonjudgmental and curious approach will facilitate patients being more forthcoming about their use. Terminology that may be familiar to regular users of cannabis such as blunts, spliffs, bowls, joints, dime bags, etc. may be unfamiliar to the provider who is performing the assessment; it is critically important to become comfortable asking follow-up questions when something is not clear, to ensure an accurate picture of the pattern of the patient's use. Patients may be able to quantify their use another way, such as in terms of money spent or amount used over a certain time period. A urine drug screen (UDS) is helpful in identifying the extent of substance use beyond solely cannabis. Also, general health and possible co-occurring mental health conditions should be assessed to differentiate between symptoms that could be attributable to other substances or other physical and mental health conditions.

**Screening, Brief Intervention, and Referral to Treatment (SBIRT) Model**

- *Screening* people helps determine their severity of cannabis use.
- *Brief interventions* use motivational interviewing to raise awareness of the consequences of use and to provide an incentive toward making positive change.
- High-risk individuals are *referred* for further assessment and *treatment.*

Screening allows the provider to assess the severity of the use in order to identify the appropriate level of treatment. Screening, brief intervention, and referral to treatment (SBIRT) is an evidence-based approach to the delivery of early intervention and treatment services to people with substance use disorders and those at risk of developing these disorders. The benefit of SBIRT is that it can be delivered in many clinical care settings. Providers should ask all patients about cannabis use, even if their use is reported as occasional and not problematic. This can also include monitoring patients for the signs and symptoms of problematic cannabis use even if use is denied by the patient. As a baseline, providers should specifically ask all patients in their practices if they have used cannabis in any form in the past year. Brief intervention focuses on increasing insight and awareness regarding substance use and motivation toward behavioral change. Brief interventions should be personalized and offered in a supportive, nonjudgmental manner. Referral to treatment provides those identified as needing more extensive treatment with access to specialty care [2].

Higher-risk groups include adolescents and young adults; patients with mood, anxiety, or psychotic disorders; and patients who use other substances. These individuals should be asked about cannabis use during routine visits, at least annually. Patients with poorly controlled chronic pain should be asked about cannabis use for analgesia. Another scenario is screening for synthetic "marijuana" products such as K2 and spice. Although these products are chemically distinct from the psychoactive compounds in the traditional cannabis plant, some cannabis users have tried synthetic "marijuana" products because of their gross physical similarity to cannabis plant matter.

A number of studies link chronic cannabis use and mental illness, and cannabis use is widespread among psychiatric patients. Effectively treating a co-occurring mental health disorder with standard treatments involving medications and behavioral therapies may help reduce cannabis use, particularly among those involved with heavy use and those with more chronic mental disorders [19, 20]. A series of large, longitudinal studies showed a link between cannabis and the development of psychosis. Use of the drug can also worsen the course of illness for patients who have schizophrenia [14]. It is not yet known to what extent cannabis is a causative agent in psychosis and to what extent it may simply exacerbate symptoms in individuals with a predisposition to psychotic symptoms. The relationship between cannabis and anxiety disorders is unsettled; while one meta-analysis showed a small positive association between cannabis use and anxiety disorders, other data has not shown this [18]. Cannabis use is common among patients with post-traumatic stress disorder (PTSD). Animal studies have found that cannabinoids can prevent stress-induced emotional and memory effects, and preliminary studies have found reduction in some PTSD symptoms in humans. There have, however, been no large-scale, controlled studies [1]. Assessing patients who use cannabis and also suffer anxiety or trauma-related disorders should be done on a case-by-case basis, with a focus on exploring the relationship of their symptoms to cannabis use.

## Treatment

Brief interventions might be useful for mild to moderate cannabis users for reducing cannabis use and/or associated consequences and have demonstrated potential for reducing cannabis use-related risk or harm indicators when compared with untreated controls [12]. There are six elements important for a brief intervention to be effective: Feedback (about personal impairment/risks), Responsibility (for change, placed on client), Advice (to change, given by clinician), Menu (of various options available, given to patient), Empathy (a style adopted by clinician), and Self-efficacy (optimistic empowerment of the client) and are commonly summarized with acronym FRAMES [11].

Psychosocial treatments of cannabinoid dependence have been tested in several studies. Supportive treatment may be provided to allow addressing underlying disorders and to aid in developing healthier coping skills when facing stressors. Motivational enhancement therapy (MET), cognitive-behavioral therapy (CBT), and contingency management (CM) have been carefully evaluated and have all shown promising results. Generally, MET is effective at engaging individuals who are ambivalent about treatment; CM can lead to longer periods of abstinence during treatment by incentivizing abstinence; and CBT can work to enhance abstinence following treatment (preventing relapse). These interventions can be delivered individually or in groups and focus on the individual or the social environment, and the focus of the therapy is to teach coping strategies and problem-solving skills [15]. Longer duration of psychotherapy is associated with better outcomes [16]. Findings also indicate that integrating all three approaches—MET, CBT, and CM—is most likely to produce positive outcomes, especially as measured by rates of abstinence from cannabis [16]. These psychosocial approaches for substance use disorders aim to build motivation, identify patterns of use and triggers that lead to use, and manage and promote substitution of substance-related behaviors with healthier activities.

Currently, there is no medication that is FDA-approved to treat cannabis use disorder, but research is active in this area and pharmacotherapy trials have been conducted as adjunctive interventions to psychosocial treatment. Studies in particular are targeting medication treatment for cannabis withdrawal symptoms; reducing or alleviating withdrawal symptoms during cessation from regular cannabis use may result in the individual being less likely to resume cannabis use and have better treatment outcomes. *N*-Acetylcysteine and gabapentin are two of the most promising medications, although no pharmacologic treatment has emerged as clearly efficacious [12]. Studies have also shown that oral THC, nabiximols, and nabilone have evidence for targeting multiple withdrawal symptoms, including cravings. Quetiapine, zolpidem, and mirtazapine may help with sleep disturbances associated with cannabis withdrawal [5].

## Conclusion

Rates of cannabis use and cannabis use disorder are on the rise in the United States resulting in an increase in number of people in need for treatment. This parallels the changes in the legal and political climate favoring legalization along with the decreased perception that cannabis use poses a significant risk of negative consequences. Screening and brief interventions can be delivered in various healthcare settings in order to identify at-risk groups and allow for treatment implantation.

Several studies have highlighted the benefit of psychosocial interventions and have concluded that a combination of CBT and MET represents the best approach to treat cannabis use disorder and that abstinence-based CM (incentives) can enhance effectiveness. Several pharmacological interventions have also been investigated; however, only a few have shown encouraging results. Future directions depend on increased research funding, greater accessibility of treatment options, and heightened awareness not only of the consequences of heavy cannabis use but the availability of specific treatments.

**Key Points**

- While many people can use cannabis use without harm, cannabis use places individuals at risk for various adverse health consequences.
- It is imperative to screen regularly for cannabis use and to characterize the use, provide education, and offer evidence-based treatments.
- Psychotherapeutic treatments, including motivational enhancement treatment (MET), cognitive-behavioral therapy (CBT), and contingency management (CM), have demonstrated effectiveness in reducing frequency and quantity of cannabis use.
- Pharmalogical treatments are targeted to decrease withdrawal symptoms. However, their effectiveness to reduce cannabis use and prevent relapse still needs further investigation.

## References


1. Abizaid A, Merali Z, Anisman H. Cannabis: a potential efficacious intervention for PTSD or simply snake oil? J Psychiatry Neurosci. 2019;44(2):75–8. https://doi.org/10.1503/jpn.190021.
2. Bernstein E, Edwards E, Dorfman D, Heeren T, Bliss C, Bernstein J. Screening and brief intervention to reduce marijuana use among youth and young adults in a pediatric emergency department. Acad Emerg Med. 2009;16(11):1174–85. https://doi.org/10.1111/j.1553-2712.2009.00490.x. PMID: 20053238; PMCID: PMC2910362.
3. Bloomfield MA, Ashok AH, Volkow ND, Howes OD. The effects of Δ9-tetrahydrocannabinol on the dopamine system. Nature. 2016;539(7629):369–77. https://doi.org/10.1038/nature20153. PMID: 27853201; PMCID: PMC5123717.
4. Bonnet U, Preuss UW. The cannabis withdrawal syndrome: current insights. Subst Abus Rehabil. 2017;8:9–37. https://doi.org/10.2147/SAR.S109576.
5. Brezing CA, Levin FR. The current state of pharmacological treatments for cannabis use disorder and withdrawal. Neuropsychopharmacology. 2018;43(1):173–94. https://doi.org/10.1038/npp.2017.212.
6. Copersino ML, Boyd SJ, Tashkin DP, Huestis MA, Heishman SJ, Dermand JC, Simmons MS, Gorelick DA. Cannabis withdrawal among non-treatment-seeking adult cannabis users. Am J Addict. 2006;15(1):8–14. https://doi.org/10.1080/10550490500418997.
7. Crean RD, Crane NA, Mason BJ. An evidence based review of acute and long-term effects of cannabis use on executive cognitive functions. J Addict Med. 2011;5(1):1–8. https://doi.org/10.1097/ADM.0b013e31820c23fa.

8. ElSohly MA, Mehmedic Z, Foster S, Gon C, Chandra S, Church JC. Changes in cannabis potency over the last two decades (1995–2014)-analysis of current data in the United States. Biol Psychiatry. 2016;79(7):613–9. https://doi.org/10.1016/j.biopsych.2016.01.004.
9. Galli JA, Sawaya RA, Friedenberg FK. Cannabinoid hyperemesis syndrome. Curr Drug Abuse Rev. 2011;4(4):241–9. https://doi.org/10.2174/1874473711104040241.
10. Marijuana Treatment Project Research Group. Brief treatments for cannabis dependence: findings from a randomized multisite trial. J Consult Clin Psychol. 2004;72(3):455–66. https://doi.org/10.1037/0022-006X.72.3.455.
11. Miller W, Sanchez V, Howard GS, Nathan PE. Motivating young adults for treatment and lifestyle. In Alcohol use and misuse by young adults, G. Howard (Ed.). University of Notre Dame Press, Notre Dame. 1993.
12. Nordstrom BR, Levin FR. Treatment of cannabis use disorders: a review of the literature. Am J Addict. 2007;16(5):331–42. https://doi.org/10.1080/10550490701525665.
13. Papaseit E, Pérez-Mañá C, Pérez-Acevedo AP, Hladun O, Torres-Moreno MC, Muga R, Torrens M, Farré M. Cannabinoids: from pot to lab. Int J Med Sci. 2018;15(12):1286–95.
14. Patel S, Khan S, Saipavankumar M, Hamid P. The association between cannabis use and schizophrenia: causative or curative? A systematic review. Cureus. 2020;12(7):e9309. https://doi.org/10.7759/cureus.9309.
15. Sabioni P, Le Foll B. Psychosocial and pharmacological interventions for the treatment of cannabis use disorder. F1000Research. 2018;7:173. https://doi.org/10.12688/f1000research.11191.1.
16. Sherman BJ, McRae-Clark AL. Treatment of cannabis use disorder: current science and future outlook. Pharmacotherapy. 2016;36:511–35.
17. Substance Abuse and Mental Health Services Administration. Key substance use and mental health indicators in the United States: results from the 2018 National Survey on Drug Use and Health (HHS Publication No. PEP19-5068, NSDUH Series H-54). Rockville: Center for Behavioral Health Statistics and Quality, Substance Abuse and Mental Health Services Administration. 2019. Retrieved from.
18. Twomey CD. Association of cannabis use with the development of elevated anxiety symptoms in the general population: a meta-analysis. J Epidemiol Community Health. 2017;71(8):811–6.
19. Volkow ND, Baler RD, Compton WM, Weiss SR. Adverse health effects of marijuana use. N Engl J Med. 2014a;370(23):2219–27.
20. Volkow ND, Baler RD, Compton WM, Weiss SR. Adverse health effects of marijuana use. N Engl J Med. 2014b;370(23):2219–27. https://doi.org/10.1056/NEJMra1402309.

# Hallucinogen-Related Disorders

5

Katherine Kim and Daniel Roberts

## Introduction

Hallucinogens comprise a diverse group of substances with differing chemical structures and mechanisms of action, but are classified together for their similar subjective effects, including alterations in perception, mood, and cognition (see Table 5.1). Many names have been proposed for this class of drugs, including *psychotomimetic* (meaning "mimicking psychosis"), *entheogen* ("bringing into being the god within"), and *psychedelic* ("mind- or soul-manifesting"). *Hallucinogen* has been its common designation in the scientific literature. However, the term *psychedelic*, which has prevailed in the lay press for decades, is increasingly the preferred term even in research settings [1, 2]. For the purposes of consistency with DSM-5 nomenclature, we use the term *hallucinogens* to refer to this group of substances in this chapter.

This diverse group of substances includes indoleamines (e.g., psilocybin, N,N-dimethyltryptamine [DMT], and the admixture ayahuasca which contains DMT), ergolines (e.g., lysergic acid diethylamide [LSD] and lysergic acid amide [LSA], which is found in morning glory seeds), phenethylamines (e.g., 3,4-methylenedioxymethamphetamine [MDMA] and mescaline), NMDA antagonists (e.g., phencyclidine [PCP] and ketamine), as well as other ethnobotanical compounds such as *Salvia divinorum* and jimsonweed [3]. Many hallucinogens are ingested orally, either swallowed as tablets, pills, or liquids; consumed raw or dried; or brewed into teas; though some can be inhaled (DMT, PCP, Salvia), snorted (ketamine, PCP), or injected (ketamine, PCP) [4].

K. Kim · D. Roberts (✉)
Department of Psychiatry, New York University School of Medicine, New York, NY, USA
e-mail: katherine.kim@nyulangone.org; dan.roberts@nyulangone.org



J. D. Avery, D. Hankins (eds.), *Addiction Medicine*, Psychiatry Update 2,
https://doi.org/10.1007/978-3-030-86430-9_5

**Table 5.1** Signs and symptoms associated with hallucinogen intoxication

| |
|---|
| Autonomic arousal (e.g., dilated pupils, hypertension, hyperthermia, gastrointestinal distress, tachycardia, tachypnea) |
| Depersonalization |
| Derealization |
| Distortions in one's sense of time |
| Ego death/dissolution (i.e., reduction in normal self-referential awareness leading to an increased feeling of unity with others and one's surroundings) |
| Mood changes (both perceived as good and bad and can be quite variable during the course of intoxication) |
| Impaired judgment |
| Impaired motor coordination |
| Mystical-type experiences |
| Perceptual changes (e.g., intensification of sensations, illusions or visual hallucinations (rarer), synesthesia) |
| Thought process changes |

**Table 5.2** Hallucinogen-related disorders (as described in the DSM-5 [3])

| |
|---|
| Phencyclidine use disorder |
| Other hallucinogen use disorder |
| Phencyclidine intoxication |
| Other hallucinogen intoxication |
| Hallucinogen persisting perception disorder |
| Other phencyclidine-induced disorders |
| Other hallucinogen-induced disorders |
| Unspecified phencyclidine-related disorder |
| Unspecified hallucinogen-related disorder |

Though a comprehensive discussion of the history of these substances is beyond the scope of this clinical text, there exists a notable history, documented on most continents, of the use of various preparations of hallucinogenic plants as part of religious and spiritual ceremonies. Substances used in this context include, but are not limited to: hallucinogenic mushrooms, used by the Aztecs and other indigenous groups from Central and North America; the DMT-containing brew ayahuasca, used by indigenous tribes in the Amazon; and mescaline-containing peyote cactus, used by indigenous peoples of Mexico and North America [5–7].

Under the category of hallucinogen-related disorders, the DSM-5 describes hallucinogen use disorders, hallucinogen-induced disorders, and acute intoxication (see Table 5.2). Although maladaptive patterns of drug use can be seen in users of PCP and ketamine, hallucinogen use disorders generally are rare, with a lifetime prevalence estimated at around 0.1–0.6% in the United States [3, 8]. Lifetime use, however, is relatively common (9.32%) [8]. Recreational use of classical hallucinogens, a group of serotonergic substances that includes LSD and psilocybin, has been found to be relatively safe from a physiologic perspective, and their use is associated with lower utilization of emergency medical treatment compared to the use of methamphetamine, cannabis, and alcohol [9–12]. Lifetime use of classical hallucinogens is not associated with the development of mental health disorders, increased rates of panic attacks, or decreased cognitive function [9].

In light of their physiological safety and their unique psychological effects, the therapeutic potential of hallucinogens has emerged as an area of clinical research [1, 2, 13]. Recent phase 1 and phase 2 clinical studies have investigated the utility of psilocybin for a number of psychiatric disorders including, but not limited to, major depressive disorder [13, 14], end-of-life psychological distress [15], and alcohol use disorder [16]; and the use of MDMA for post-traumatic stress disorder [17]. Moreover, research over the last 10 years has established a substantial evidence base for the therapeutic utility of ketamine in the treatment of acute suicidal ideation [18] as well as unipolar and bipolar depression [19]. Although thought to be physically safe for consumption for most adults, hallucinogens cause a temporary disruption to ordinary mind states, which, for some, can cause psychological distress during the experience. Other adverse effects can include physiological toxicity, physiological tolerance, and prolonged psychopathology [20], which we explore in the case examples below.

Clinicians may encounter patients presenting with either acute intoxication or complications related to hallucinogen use. Acute hallucinogen intoxication may present with symptoms that overlap to some extent with endogenous manic, psychotic, or dissociative states. Other conditions that may cause hallucinations, delusions, and cognitive impairment, such as traumatic brain injury, delirium, and acute mania, psychosis, or dissociation, should also be considered. A history of recent consumption of a hallucinogenic substance, as well as what is typically the very transient nature of these presenting symptoms, should help to clarify the diagnosis. In making the diagnosis of hallucinogen intoxication, other conditions that may cause hallucinations, delusions, and cognitive impairment, such as traumatic brain injury, delirium, and acute mania, psychosis, or dissociation, should also be considered. Severe adverse effects and fatalities associated with hallucinogens are usually due to illicit drug impurities and/or coingestion of other drugs or alcohol [21].

The cases outlined in this chapter depict a variety of clinical scenarios related to the use of hallucinogens. They illustrate a comprehensive approach to treatment, including the stabilization of patients in the acute phase of intoxication with supportive psychological interventions. Should such an intervention fail to relieve the acute distress, psychopharmacological interventions can be used. We also discuss how to meet the long-term needs of patients with hallucinogen-related disorders, including the management of potential complications, and counseling patients in ongoing treatment.

## Clinical Cases

### Case 1

Angel is a 32-year-old man brought to the emergency room (ER) by emergency medical services (EMS) with a police escort after being agitated in public, where he had been yelling at passersby and attempting to fight with police officers when approached. This is his fifth visit in the past six months under similar circumstances. The clinical impression in his prior visits had been acute intoxication of various substances, including PCP, which was occasionally confirmed by urine toxicology when Angel was more agreeable to diagnostic workup. On initial assessment at triage, Angel is oddly related, paranoid, and endorses various delusions. His heart rate and blood pressure are elevated, and he has prominent nystagmus. Shortly into the triage process, while awaiting assessment in the busy ER milieu, Angel becomes increasingly agitated and verbally threatening. Despite the staff's efforts at verbal de-escalation, he begins swinging his fists at them and ultimately requires intramuscular medication and physical restraints to ensure safety.

### Discussion

Angel is presenting with signs of altered mental status, paranoid ideation, delusional thoughts, autonomic hyperactivity, nystagmus, and acute aggression. Given his history of similar clinical presentations, many of which objectively confirmed recent PCP use, phencyclidine intoxication is high on the differential diagnosis (see Table 5.3). This diagnosis is made based upon the history and clinical evaluation. However, because a clear history can be difficult to obtain in these circumstances, a

**Table 5.3** Phencyclidine intoxication diagnostic criteria (excerpt from the DSM-5 [3])

| |
|---|
| A. Recent use of phencyclidine (or a pharmacologically similar substance). |
| B. Clinically significant problematic behavioral changes (e.g., belligerence, assaultiveness, impulsiveness, unpredictability, psychomotor agitation, impaired judgment) that developed during, or shortly after, phencyclidine use. |
| C. Within 1 hour, two (or more) of the following signs or symptoms:<br>*Note*: When the drug is smoked, "snorted," or used intravenously, the onset may be particularly rapid.<br>1. Vertical or horizontal nystagmus.<br>2. Hypertension or tachycardia.<br>3. Numbness or diminished responsiveness to pain.<br>4. Ataxia.<br>5. Dysarthria.<br>6. Muscle rigidity.<br>7. Seizures or coma.<br>8. Hyperacusis. |
| D. The signs or symptoms are not attributable to another medical condition and are not better explained by another mental disorder, including intoxication with another substance |

working diagnosis must suffice until safety has been established and the altered mental status and impulsive, dangerous behavior have improved.

Other etiologies that might present with similar symptoms include substance withdrawal from alcohol or benzodiazepines, toxidromes, or infections (such as encephalitis, meningitis, or sepsis), particularly given the combination of altered mental status and vital sign abnormalities. Metabolic abnormalities that may cause altered mental status, including hypoglycemia, hyponatremia, or hyperthyroidism, as well as seizure disorders and vascular pathologies, should also be ruled out with the appropriate medical workup. Additionally, given the variable symptoms associated with intoxication, and because both intentional and unintentional coingestion of multiple substances are common, the differential diagnosis should include intoxication with other psychoactive substances, including not only those commonly presenting with agitation and altered mental status (e.g., amphetamines, cocaine), but also novel psychoactive substances, particularly given the growing online market for various synthetic ("designer") drugs, most of which cannot be detected on standard urine drug screens.

As the DSM-5 points out, the combination of nystagmus, elevated heart rate and/or blood pressure, and bizarre and aggressive behavior often helps to distinguish PCP intoxication from intoxication due to other substances, particularly other hallucinogens. Urine toxicology may be useful in the diagnostic workup, especially in a setting that allows for extended observation, where a clinician might have the benefit of longitudinal observation to distinguish between a short-term, substance-induced etiology and a primary psychotic or affective illness that warrants hospital admission. With respect to diagnostic workup, PCP is detectable in the urine, but may be detected up to approximately 8 days after use, so its presence is not necessarily diagnostic. Other common laboratory abnormalities associated with PCP intoxication include an elevated creatine kinase (CK or CPK) and elevated hepatic transaminases [3]. As noted above, if clinical suspicion for a medical etiology is high, then the appropriate laboratory tests should also be performed.

In this particular case example, Angel is presenting as paranoid with delusional content, and so, per the DSM-5, an additional diagnosis of phencyclidine-induced psychotic disorder should be considered in a patient presenting with the symptoms of PCP intoxication with the noted absence of intact reality testing. Moreover, a review of Angel's history, particularly his repeated presentations and continued use of PCP despite consequences within a 12-month period, suggests that phencyclidine use disorder should also be considered.

As noted in the case introduction, Angel's behavior quickly escalated to the point of serious concern for safety to both staff and the patient. In cases of PCP intoxication with agitation, particularly in busy medical settings, a supportive approach to reduce agitation would include efforts to reduce external stimulation, for example, by placing the patient in a darker, quieter space that still allows for adequate monitoring. Offering a patient a benzodiazepine, particularly in a quiet, calm, environment, can be an effective strategy that may eliminate the need for involuntary medication and/or physical restraints. However, if these measures are unavailable or ineffective, and patient or staff safety is at risk, safe and efficient symptom reduction is essential.

Physical restraints may be initially necessary to safely administer sedating medications. Safe and effective physical restraint may require several staff members, given PCP's propensity to cause both significant activation and reduced perception of pain.

Based upon observational reports and clinical experience, antipsychotics and/or benzodiazepines are often the preferred types of sedating agents. Regarding benzodiazepines, general clinical consensus recommends lorazepam 4 mg intravenously (IV) or midazolam 5 mg IV, or by intramuscular (IM) injection if IV access is not available [22]. Regarding antipsychotics, droperidol 2.5 mg or haloperidol 5 mg IM or IV can be used as adjunctive therapy if benzodiazepines do not adequately control symptoms [22]. These doses may be repeated until adequate sedation is achieved to establish safety. In reviewing the literature, there is some anecdotal caution to avoid antipsychotics such as droperidol or haloperidol due to the potential concern of lowering a patient's seizure threshold or that these agents may impair heat dissipation in patients experiencing hyperthermia. However, there do not appear to be any high-quality human studies to support these claims, and significant clinical experience suggests that antipsychotics or the coadministration with benzodiazepines can be safely utilized.

Clinicians should be aware of multiple serious complications that can occur with PCP intoxication and the attendant behaviors, particularly with ingestion of large quantities of PCP. These include rhabdomyolysis, seizures, hypoglycemia, trauma, and coma. Any patient with such significant complications should be triaged to an appropriate medical setting and likely requires admission to an intensive care setting for monitoring and treatment.

Given the variable presentation of PCP toxicity and the potentially problematic behavioral issues associated with intoxication, most patients presenting in the emergency setting benefit from observation. The intoxication period from PCP usually lasts for several hours, so a patient presenting early following ingestion could quickly escalate in terms of problematic behaviors and safety concerns, and so should be retained in an appropriate setting where they can be safely monitored while metabolizing any ingested substances. Of note, in individuals with a co-occurring mental illness, other substance use disorders, genetic loading for mental illness, or other psychiatric or behavioral vulnerabilities, the hallucinogenic effects of PCP may last beyond the typical time period and may precipitate a persistent psychotic episode resembling schizophrenia spectrum illness.

PCP use disorder is defined by the same criteria as other substance use disorders in the DSM-5. The use of motivational interviewing can be helpful in assisting patients to become aware of and resolving ambivalence of decreasing or stopping PCP use [23]. One large study found the incidence of PCP intoxication-related injuries to be 13%, with self-inflicted injuries representing 22% of those [24]. As such, when counseling active PCP users, a harm-reduction approach that emphasizes the maintenance of physical safety is important. Although pharmacological treatments for any co-occurring substance use or psychiatric disorders may be helpful in this patient population, there are no FDA-approved treatments for PCP use disorder. However, enrollment in outpatient counseling or inpatient rehabilitation centers may be helpful in patients who are motivated for treatment. Additionally, 12-step support programs are a widely available and free community resource that may assist in supporting abstinence.

## Case 2

Phil is a 22-year-old man that comes into the ER accompanied by his friend, who informs staff that the patient had ingested some "shrooms" a couple hours earlier with a group of friends. The friend notes that shortly thereafter, Phil became acutely anxious and paranoid. He reported visions of frightening figures on the wall and began repeatedly announcing that the "world is corrupt." Given his level of distress, he asked his friend to take him to the ER. During the assessment, Phil is able to provide a narrative of the day's events and his mushroom ingestion, but he appears anxious and guarded and states that he is afraid that these experiences and feelings will never go away. His heart rate and blood pressure are elevated, and his pupils appear dilated. He responds to verbal reassurance and is taken to a quiet room, where he is offered medications, which appear to calm him. Some hours later, after a subjective report of improvement in symptoms and apparent return to his physical, cognitive, and psychological baseline, he is discharged from the ER.

One month later, Phil presents to his primary care doctor complaining of visual abnormalities, including visual trailing, spontaneous flashes of color, and illusory palinopsia (a persistence of a visual image after the stimulus has been removed). He reports that he has not used any substances since his ER visit.

## Discussion

At his initial visit, Phil is presenting with the acute onset of significant psychological changes (e.g., marked anxiety, fear of losing control, and paranoia), alterations in sensory perception, and abnormal vital signs following ingestion of presumed psilocybin-containing mushrooms. His signs and symptoms meet the DSM-5 diagnostic criteria for other hallucinogen intoxication.

The overall effect of any psychoactive drug is a complex interaction of many elements beyond direct pharmacological mechanisms, including physiological, psychological, cultural, and environmental factors [20]. Although we assess for the influence of these factors with any patient, they may have an especially important role in the experience of a person who has ingested a hallucinogenic compound. A group of influences in this context has been collectively termed "set and setting." "Set" refers to individual factors such as one's mindset, personality structure, and expectations; "setting" includes environmental factors, such as the physical location, the situation, and the cultural context in which the hallucinogen use occurs. These elements are thought to underlie the differences in emotional valence, level of anxiety, and overall experience of different users at different times despite ingesting the same substance. Colloquially, the subjective experience of acute intoxication is referred to as a "trip," and a "bad trip" refers to those experiences predominantly marked by anxiety, dysphoria, fear, or agitation. Neuropsychiatric effects occur in response to administration of any hallucinogen, and although the various substances (e.g., LSD versus MDMA) differ in their onset, duration, and intensity of effects, their acute psychological and behavioral symptoms can be quite similar (see Table 5.1).

As in both Angel's and Phil's cases, many hallucinogens produce sympathomimetic effects such as dilated pupils, elevations in blood pressure and heart rate, and, on rare occasions, hyperthermia. The DSM-5 requires at least two physiologic signs, in addition to psychological and perceptual changes, to meet diagnostic criteria for other hallucinogen intoxication (in this case, with psilocybin). Though mild vital sign fluctuations can occur with psilocybin intoxication, significant vital sign abnormalities are uncommon and should prompt consideration of another intoxicant (e.g., PCP, amphetamines, or cocaine) or other medical etiologies. Hyperthermia rarely occurs with isolated hallucinogen intoxication, and this is a sign of severe toxicity. It can also be a sign of serotonin toxicity ("serotonin syndrome"), a condition characterized by the presence of altered mental status, neuromuscular abnormalities, and autonomic hyperactivity that typically occurs in the setting of coingestion of serotonergic hallucinogens (e.g., LSD, MDMA, or psilocybin) and other serotonergic medications such as antidepressants (e.g., SSRIs or MAOIs), analgesics (e.g., meperidine), antiemetics (e.g., ondansetron), or herbal supplements (e.g., St. John's wort). A patient presenting with signs and symptoms concerning for serotonin syndrome, especially with hyperthermia, should be promptly triaged to an appropriate medical setting and likely requires admission to an intensive care setting for monitoring and treatment.

Of note, most patients presenting with hallucinogen intoxication are awake and oriented, are able to provide a coherent history of preceding events including hallucinogen use, and have good insight that their symptoms are substance-induced. These patients, in the absence of severe symptoms, typically do not require, nor benefit, from routine laboratory tests, especially given the fact that most hallucinogens are not detectable on routine urine toxicology screens. However, the presence of altered mental status, overt psychosis (especially with auditory hallucinations), severe agitation, or bizarre behavior should prompt further medical workup to rule out other medical etiologies [25].

In most cases of intoxication, supportive care is all that is needed to manage a patient's distress. The general clinical consensus suggests embracing a nondirective and nonconfrontational approach while allowing the patient to relax in a calming environment until the substance's effects subside. In Phil's case, he was offered medications in the ER, which is often done. Psychopharmacological interventions, such as benzodiazepines and/or antipsychotics, are generally only necessary if there is concern for the safety of the patient or others. Some clinicians who have had significant experience in working with patients having difficult psychological experiences while intoxicated from hallucinogens have cautioned that pharmacologically terminating a "bad trip" can potentially have a negative psychological impact on a patient [25, 26], although this has not been explored in clinical trials.

Most cases of other hallucinogen intoxication are time-limited and resolve over the course of several hours, ultimately resulting in a patient returning to their neuropsychiatric baseline and being able to leave the ER without residual symptoms or complications. However, in the case of Phil, he began to experience some distressing symptoms some weeks later, consistent with the unique disorder of hallucinogen persisting perception disorder (HPPD).

## Hallucinogen Persisting Perception Disorder (HPPD)

HPPD is a relatively rare and poorly understood phenomenon, with anecdotal reports associating this diagnosis primarily, though not exclusively, with LSD use [3]. HPPD is described in the DSM-5 as the reexperiencing of one or more perceptual symptoms after cessation of hallucinogen use. Of note, these perceptual disturbances may not have been experienced during the acute intoxication experience, a period typically not lasting more than several hours maximum [27]. Visual symptoms can include geometric hallucinations, false perceptions of movement in the peripheral visual fields, flashes or intensification of colors, trailing images of moving objects, positive afterimages, halos around objects, and misperceptions of relative size (macropsia, micropsia). HPPD may co-occur with dissociative phenomena. The symptoms can emerge after one-time use or at any point after more frequent use and may be experienced episodically or persistently [28]. The symptoms can begin after a latent period of days to months or even years, and they may last for months to years. Interestingly, without treatment, both spontaneous improvement and persistent symptoms have been reported [29, 30].

HPPD is a diagnosis of exclusion. Patients need to be carefully evaluated for other causes of perceptual disturbances, such as anatomical brain lesions and central nervous system infections, seizure disorders, migraines, head trauma, hypnopompic/hypnagogic hallucinations, delirium, major neurocognitive disorders, primary psychotic disorders, substance intoxication, and substance-induced psychotic disorders. Given the relatively low incidence of HPPD, a neurological evaluation that includes an EEG and brain MRI may be warranted to rule out neurological causes. In addition to ruling out psychiatric disorders that may better explain the visual symptoms, screening for concurrent psychiatric comorbidities such as depression, anxiety, panic disorder, and psychotic disorders is critical, as HPPD can cause significant distress and clinical impairment. As with any psychiatric presentation, the patient should also be assessed for suicidality [31].

Counseling provided to patients with HPPD should include recommendations to avoid further use of hallucinogens and to limit the use of other substances. Assessment of the triggers for visual symptoms may prevent further exacerbation. The use of motivational interviewing may be helpful in those who, despite persisting symptoms of HPPD, appear unmotivated or ambivalent around the recommendation to limit their use of hallucinogenic substances [23]. Educating patients on the possible outcomes of HPPD, which include spontaneous remission or persistent symptoms with unpredictable frequency and intensity, can be helpful in managing expectations. To this end, psychotherapeutic interventions, including the use of mindfulness- and acceptance-based psychotherapies, may also be helpful. Cognitive-behavioral approaches can also be used to target any distorted cognitions, depression, and/or anxiety that might occur secondary to HPPD symptoms.

Lastly, judicious use of psychotropic medications may be of some utility in patients whose symptoms cause persistent and clinically significant distress despite non-pharmacologic therapies. However, given the paucity of data regarding efficacy of psychotropic medications in HPPD and the possibility of spontaneous remission, a thorough discussion of the risks and benefits of pharmacologic treatment is particularly important in these cases. Open-label studies and case reports suggest possible benefit from treatment with benzodiazepines, anticonvulsants, and alpha-2-agonists, while results from studies of selective serotonin reuptake inhibitors (SSRIs) and antipsychotics are mixed. Among the latter, risperidone appears to worsen symptoms [32, 33]. However, given the low prevalence of HPPD, a meaningful interpretation of these findings is limited by a very small sample size. Given the potential side effects of medications, a shorter course of treatment should be considered; however, the risk of rebound symptoms after withdrawing such treatment has not been studied.

## Integration

It is worth emphasizing that, although hallucinogen intoxication is generally an acute, time-limited experience that does not result in chronic adverse effects and hallucinogen use disorders are rare, these experiences can be very challenging and cause significant psychological distress that can leave a person feeling unsettled for some time after the acute intoxication has resolved. Additionally, even the visions and insights one may experience during a so-called "good trip" can be challenging to understand, and it can be difficult to incorporate these experiences into one's daily life. In response to this perceived need, there is a growing number of licensed mental health clinicians that offer ongoing psychotherapeutic services, often referred to as "Psychedelic Integration Therapy," focused on providing psychoeducation, and to help individuals process and integrate their experiences with hallucinogens.

The resurgence of scientific research focused on hallucinogen-assisted psychotherapy has generated significant positive media coverage in the recent years. As a result, it is possible that there may be an increase in the number of individuals that decide to experiment with hallucinogens. Future studies will likely focus on how to optimize experiences with hallucinogens, and, in particular, explore if, how, and to what extent integration work factors into the overall positive results observed in recent hallucinogen-assisted psychotherapy studies. Given the increased awareness of these substances and the potential for growing prevalence and incidence of use, it will be important for clinicians to be able to provide accurate psychoeducation about these substances and for there to be resources that can offer appropriate psychotherapeutic support for patients in need.

## Case 3

Sasha is a 21-year-old woman who was brought to the emergency department by EMS after being found unconscious at a dance club. She is accompanied by a friend who reported that Sasha had used "Molly" and ketamine during the course of the evening. On physical exam, the patient appears lethargic. Vital signs are notable for mild hypertension and tachycardia. Neurologic exam showed no signs of myoclonus, hyperreflexia, nystagmus, or tremor. Laboratory results show a mild hyponatremia but are otherwise within normal limits. Sasha was admitted to the inpatient medicine service for monitoring and supportive treatment with IV fluids, which corrected her hyponatremia, and her vital signs and mental status normalized. Now returned to baseline, she is discharged home shortly thereafter.

## Discussion

MDMA ("Molly" or "Ecstasy") and ketamine are commonly used in the recreational setting, where they are often referred to as "club drugs." MDMA has both hallucinogenic and stimulant-like properties and is used to achieve these and other effects, including a sense of tranquility, euphoria, and increased emotional openness and empathy. Ketamine, which has FDA approval for use as an anesthetic agent, is also used recreationally, as subanesthetic doses induce prominent dissociative and hallucinogenic effects. Like PCP, MDMA and ketamine may have higher abuse potential compared to other hallucinogens [34, 35].

Acute treatment of MDMA and/or ketamine intoxication begins with medical assessment and stabilization, given the potential complications of unmonitored use. Adverse effects of acute MDMA intoxication are well established. MDMA intoxication may cause acute hypertension, tachycardia, and/or hyperthermia. Cardiac complications of MDMA intoxication can include hypertensive emergencies, arrhythmias, heart failure, and myocardial infarction [36]. Hyperthermia may be caused by direct drug effects on the central nervous system, as well as from physical exertion or environmental conditions, and can be lethal. As such, these patients may require rapid cooling to stabilize their temperature and to mitigate downstream adverse effects, including rhabdomyolysis, myoglobinuria, renal failure, and disseminated intravascular coagulopathy, among others [37, 38].

In a patient with autonomic instability, altered cognition, and symptoms of myoclonus, hyperreflexia, or tremor, there should be a high suspicion for serotonin syndrome (see Case 2 above for details regarding serotonin toxicity). In addition to serotonin syndrome, hyponatremia may occur in intoxicated patients (as it did in Sasha's case). This is largely the result of increased fluid intake due to the polydipsia that is commonly caused by MDMA, though syndrome of inappropriate antidiuretic hormone (SIADH) may also contribute. Significant hyponatremia can lead to nausea, malaise, encephalopathy, seizures, and death [39]. Hepatotoxicity is another possible adverse effect, and laboratory values should be closely monitored [40]. Patients who present to the emergency room with complications of acute MDMA intoxication may require admission to the hospital for appropriate monitoring and treatment.

Various authors have proposed that environmental or behavioral factors surrounding MDMA use likely play more of a contributory role in the development of reported adverse events, such as vigorous dancing or physical activity, inadvertent disregard of physical cues, and excessive or reduced hydration resulting in hyperthermia or hyponatremia [41]. There has also been much concern raised through the years in the lay press, as well as by some researchers, about the potential neurotoxic effects of MDMA in humans [42, 43]; however subsequent reviews of these initial reports with follow-up analyses have countered that the concerning claims are based on animal studies that included unrealistically high doses of MDMA and on human studies comparing repeated use of MDMA, often concurrently with other substances [41, 44, 45]. This debate is ongoing, but from growing studies including MDMA-assisted psychotherapy, it does not appear that cognitive function is negatively impacted [41, 44, 45].

Like MDMA, ketamine can be used in the recreational setting, either alone or in combination with other drugs. At higher doses (like those used in anesthesia), it can suppress consciousness or induce coma. However, in smaller doses, it can cause reduced alertness, altered sensory perception, ataxia, cognitive impairment, and mild increases in heart rate and blood pressure [34]. Nystagmus can be seen but is less common than that seen in PCP intoxication. Chronic use can lead to urologic injury including ketamine-induced ulcerative cystitis, with symptoms of increased frequency and urgency of urination, dysuria, urge incontinence, and hematuria, and which may be irreversible even after cessation of use [46]. Frequent ketamine use can also be rarely associated with hydronephrosis or papillary necrosis [46]. Abdominal pain is a common complaint among chronic, heavy users of ketamine and may be associated with liver injury [46, 47]. Like with MDMA, chronic use of ketamine may also lead to cognitive deficits [48].

As with other substance use disorders, enrolling in an outpatient treatment program or inpatient rehabilitation center may be helpful for patients who want to decrease or stop use. Psychotherapeutic interventions including motivational interviewing can help patients understand the role that substance use plays in their lives [23]. Psychoeducation on adverse consequences may help patients recognize and seek help for any medical complications of their use; it is especially important for patients to be able to recognize life-threatening conditions such as malignant hyperthermia and serotonin syndrome. Pharmacologically, there are no FDA-approved treatments for hallucinogen use disorders. Pharmacological treatments for co-occurring substance use disorders, as well as treatment of any psychiatric comorbidities, may likely be helpful in these patients. And, as discussed above in Angel's case, 12-step support programs are a widely available and free community resource that may assist in supporting one's desire for abstinence.

## Conclusion

In this chapter, we discussed scenarios clinicians may encounter with patients presenting with hallucinogen-related disorders. In acute intoxication of most hallucinogens (not including PCP), supportive care is often all that is needed to manage a patient's time-limited distress while waiting for the substance to metabolize over the typical course of several hours. Patients typically return to their neuropsychiatric and physical baseline without any residual symptoms or complications. However, acute PCP intoxication can present with altered mental status and bizarre and aggressive behavior that puts the patient and others at serious risk of harm, and so this condition often requires pharmacological intervention and continued observation. Additionally, it is imperative for patients presenting with altered mental status or severe vital sign abnormalities to be assessed for medical complications and to be triaged to the appropriate medical setting including an intensive care unit if appropriate. In the outpatient setting, being able to provide psychoeducation and harm reduction strategies for patients may also be useful, including education on the complications of chronic use of hallucinogens. In general, pharmacological treatments are limited for hallucinogen use disorders, but assessment and treatment of co-occurring substance use disorders and other psychiatric disorders are important. Outpatient substance use settings, community-based 12-step support groups, and inpatient rehabilitation programs may be helpful for patients who are struggling, but motivated, to decrease or abstain from use of hallucinogens.

### Key Points

- Hallucinogens comprise a diverse group of substances with differing chemical structures and mechanisms of action but are classified together for producing similar subjective alterations in perception, mood, and cognition and for producing altered states of consciousness.
- Maladaptive patterns of drug use can be seen with PCP and ketamine, but hallucinogen use disorders, in general, are rare.
- PCP intoxication can produce significant medical complications and unpredictable neuropsychiatric symptoms that place both the patient and others at risk of harm and may warrant proper medical workup and observation with appropriate treatment to minimize serious complications and safety risks.
- "Set" (individual factors) and "setting" (environmental factors) can greatly impact one's overall experience with hallucinogens.
- Distress associated with other hallucinogen intoxication is often time-limited and can be generally managed with supportive care.
- There is a resurgence of scientific research focused on hallucinogens and hallucinogen-assisted psychotherapy, with numerous positive preliminary reports including safety and tolerability in targeting various psychiatric conditions, but there is much still to be learned about this class of substances.

- There are growing numbers of licensed mental health clinicians and facilities that offer psychotherapeutic services for individuals seeking assistance in processing and integrating difficult experiences with hallucinogens.

## References


1. Nichols DE. Hallucinogens. Pharmacol Ther. 2004;101(2):131–81. https://doi.org/10.1016/j.pharmthera.2003.11.002.
2. Reiff CM, Richman EE, Nemeroff CB, Carpenter LL, Widge AS, Rodriguez CI, Work Group on Biomarkers and Novel Treatments, a Division of the American Psychiatric Association Council of Research. Psychedelics and psychedelic-assisted psychotherapy. Am J Psychiatr. 2020;177(5):391–410.
3. American Psychiatric Association. Diagnostic and statistical manual of mental disorders. 5th ed. 2013. https://doi.org/10.1176/appi.books.9780890425596.
4. National Institute on Drug Abuse. (2020, July 6). Hallucinogens DrugFacts. https://www.drugabuse.gov/publications/drugfacts/hallucinogens.
5. Carod-Artal FJ. Hallucinogenic drugs in pre-Columbian Mesoamerican cultures. Neurologia (Barcelona, Spain). 2015;30(1):42–9. https://doi.org/10.1016/j.nrl.2011.07.003.
6. Araújo AM, Carvalho F, de Lourdes Bastos M, de Pinho PG, Carvalho M. The hallucinogenic world of tryptamines: an updated review. Arch Toxicol. 2015;89(8):1151–73. https://doi.org/10.1007/s00204-015-1513-x.
7. Schultes RE, Hofmann A, Rätsch C. Plants of the gods: their sacred, healing and hallucinogenic powers. 2nd ed. Rochester: Inner Traditions; 2006.
8. Shalit N, Rehm J, Lev-Ran S. Epidemiology of hallucinogen use in the U.S. results from the national epidemiologic survey on alcohol and related conditions III. Addict Behav. 2019;89:35–43. https://doi.org/10.1016/j.addbeh.2018.09.020.
9. Nutt DJ, King LA, Phillips LD. Drug harms in the UK: a multicriteria decision analysis. Lancet. 2010;376(9752):1558–65.
10. Castellanos JP, Woolley C, Bruno KA, Zeidan F, Halberstadt A, Furnish T. Chronic pain and psychedelics: a review and proposed mechanism of action. Reg Anesth Pain Med. 2020;45(7):486–94.
11. Griffiths RR, Richards WA, McCann U, Jesse R. Psilocybin can occasion mystical-type experiences having substantial and sustained personal meaning and spiritual significance. Psychopharmacology. 2006;187(3):268–92. https://doi.org/10.1007/s00213-006-0457-5.
12. Grob CS, Danforth AL, Chopra GS, Hagerty M, McKay CR, Halberstadt AL, Greer GR. Pilot study of psilocybin treatment for anxiety in patients with advanced-stage cancer. Arch Gen Psychiatry. 2011;68(1):71–8. https://doi.org/10.1001/archgenpsychiatry.2010.116.
13. Carhart-Harris RL, Goodwin GM. The therapeutic potential of psychedelic drugs: past, present, and future. Neuropsychopharmacology. 2017;42(11):2105–13. https://doi.org/10.1038/npp.2017.84.
14. Davis AK, Barrett FS, May DG, Cosimano MP, Sepeda ND, Johnson MW, Finan PH, Griffiths RR. Effects of psilocybin-assisted therapy on major depressive disorder: a randomized clinical trial. JAMA Psychiat. 2020; https://doi.org/10.1001/jamapsychiatry.2020.3285.
15. Ross S, Bossis A, Guss J, Agin-Liebes G, Malone T, Cohen B, et al. Rapid and sustained symptom reduction following psilocybin treatment for anxiety and depression in patients with life-threatening cancer: a randomized controlled trial. J Psychopharmacol. 2016;30(12):1165–80.
16. Bogenschutz MP, Forcehimes AA, Pommy JA, Wilcox CE, Barbosa PCR, Strassman RJ. Psilocybin-assisted treatment for alcohol dependence: a proof-of-concept study. J Psychopharmacol (Oxford, England). 2015;29(3):289–99. https://doi.org/10.1177/0269881114565144.

17. Mithoefer MC, Feduccia AA, Jerome L, Mithoefer A, Wagner M, Walsh Z, Hamilton S, Yazar-Klosinski B, Emerson A, Doblin R. MDMA-assisted psychotherapy for treatment of PTSD: study design and rationale for phase 3 trials based on pooled analysis of six phase 2 randomized controlled trials. Psychopharmacology. 2019;236(9):2735–45. https://doi.org/10.1007/s00213-019-05249-5.
18. Wilkinson ST, Ballard ED, Bloch MH, Mathew SJ, Murrough JW, Feder A, Sos P, Wang G, Zarate CA, Sanacora G. The effect of a single dose of intravenous ketamine on suicidal ideation: a systematic review and individual participant data meta-analysis. Am J Psychiatry. 2018;175(2):150–8. https://doi.org/10.1176/appi.ajp.2017.17040472.
19. Lee EE, Della Selva MP, Liu A, Himelhoch S. Ketamine as a novel treatment for major depressive disorder and bipolar depression: a systematic review and quantitative meta-analysis. Gen Hosp Psychiatry. 2015;37(2):178–84. https://doi.org/10.1016/j.genhosppsych.2015.01.003.
20. Addy PH, D'Souza D. Hallucinogen use disorders. In: Ebert MH, Leckman JF, Petrakis IL, editors. Current diagnosis & treatment: psychiatry. 3rd ed. McGraw-Hill; 2019. https://accessmedicine.mhmedical.com/content.aspx?bookid=2509&sectionid=200980991.
21. van Amsterdam J, Opperhuizen A, van den Brink W. Harm potential of magic mushroom use: a review. Regul Toxicol Pharmacol. 2011;59(3):423–9. https://doi.org/10.1016/j.yrtph.2011.01.006.
22. Heard, K., & Hoppe, J. (2020). Phencyclidine (PCP) intoxication in adults. In Traub SJ, Grayzel J, editors. UpToDate. https://www.uptodate.com/contents/phencyclidine-pcp-intoxication-in-adults?search=pcp%20intoxication&source=search_result&selectedTitle=1~21&usage_type=default&display_rank=1#H17.
23. DiClemente CC, Corno CM, Graydon MM, Wiprovnick AE, Knoblach DJ. Motivational interviewing, enhancement, and brief interventions over the last decade: a review of reviews of efficacy and effectiveness. Psychol Addict Behav. 2017;31(8):862–87. https://doi.org/10.1037/adb0000318.
24. McCarron MM, Schulze BW, Thompson GA, Conder MC, Goetz WA. Acute phencyclidine intoxication: incidence of clinical findings in 1,000 cases. Ann Emerg Med. 1981;10(5):237–42. https://doi.org/10.1016/s0196-0644(81)80047-9.
25. Grof C, Grof S. Spiritual emergency: the understanding and treatment of transpersonal crises. Int J Transpers Stud. 2017;36(2) https://doi.org/10.24972/ijts.2017.36.2.30.
26. Viggiano DB, Krippner S. The Grofs' model of spiritual emergency in retrospect: has it stood the test of time? Int J Transpers Stud. 2010;29(1):118–27.
27. Lerner AG, Goodman C, Rudinski D, Lev-Ran S. LSD flashbacks – the appearance of new visual imagery not experienced during initial intoxication: two case reports. Isr J Psychiatry Relat Sci. 2014a;51(4):307–9.
28. Halpern JH, Lerner AG, Passie T. A review of Hallucinogen Persisting Perception Disorder (HPPD) and an exploratory study of subjects claiming symptoms of HPPD. Curr Top Behav Neurosci. 2018;36:333–60. https://doi.org/10.1007/7854_2016_457.
29. Hermle L, Simon M, Ruchsow M, Geppert M. Hallucinogen-persisting perception disorder. Ther Adv Psychopharmacol. 2012;2(5):199–205. https://doi.org/10.1177/2045125312451270.
30. Abraham HD, Duffy FH. EEG coherence in post-LSD visual hallucinations. Psychiatry Res. 2001;107(3):151–63. https://doi.org/10.1016/s0925-4927(01)00098-1.
31. Brodrick J, Mitchell BG. Hallucinogen persisting perception disorder and risk of suicide. J Pharm Pract. 2016;29(4):431–4. https://doi.org/10.1177/0897190014566314.
32. Lerner GA, Rudinski D, Bor O, Goodman C. Flashbacks and HPPD: a clinical-oriented concise review. Isr J Psychiatry Relat Sci. 2014;51(4):296–301.
33. Martinotti G, Santacroce R, Pettorruso M, Montemitro C, Spano MC, Lorusso M, di Giannantonio M, Lerner AG. Hallucinogen persisting perception disorder: etiology, clinical features, and therapeutic perspectives. Brain Sci. 2018;8(3) https://doi.org/10.3390/brainsci8030047.
34. Liu Y, Lin D, Wu B, Zhou W. Ketamine abuse potential and use disorder. Brain Res Bull. 2016;126(Pt 1):68–73. https://doi.org/10.1016/j.brainresbull.2016.05.016.

35. Aarde SM, Taffe MA. Predicting the abuse liability of Entactogen-class, new and emerging psychoactive substances via preclinical models of drug self-administration. Curr Top Behav Neurosci. 2017;32:145–64. https://doi.org/10.1007/7854_2016_54.
36. Shenouda SK, Carvalho F, Varner KJ. The cardiovascular and cardiac actions of ecstasy and its metabolites. Curr Pharm Biotechnol. 2010;11(5):470–5. https://doi.org/10.2174/138920110791591526.
37. Callaway CW, Clark RF. Hyperthermia in psychostimulant overdose. Ann Emerg Med. 1994;24(1):68–76. https://doi.org/10.1016/s0196-0644(94)70165-2.
38. Kalant H. The pharmacology and toxicology of "ecstasy" (MDMA) and related drugs. CMAJ. 2001;165(7):917–28.
39. Hartung TK, Schofield E, Short AI, Parr MJA, Henry JA. Hyponatraemic states following 3,4-methylenedioxymethamphetamine (MDMA, 'ecstasy') ingestion. QJM. 2002;95(7):431–7. https://doi.org/10.1093/qjmed/95.7.431.
40. Carvalho M, Pontes H, Remião F, Bastos ML, Carvalho F. Mechanisms underlying the hepatotoxic effects of ecstasy. Curr Pharm Biotechnol. 2010;11(5):476–95. https://doi.org/10.2174/138920110791591535.
41. Multidisciplinary Association For Psychedelic Studies (MAPS). MDMA Investigator's Brochure. 2020, August 17. https://mapscontent.s3-us-west-1.amazonaws.com/research-archive/MDMA+IB+12th+Edition+Final+17AUG2020.pdf.
42. Ricaurte GA, DeLanney LE, Irwin I, Langston JW. Toxic effects of MDMA on central serotonergic neurons in the primate: importance of route and frequency of drug administration. Brain Res. 1988;446(1):165–8.
43. Boot BP, McGregor IS, Hall W. MDMA (ecstasy) neurotoxicity: assessing and communicating the risks. Lancet (London, England). 2000;355(9217):1818–21. https://doi.org/10.1016/S0140-6736(00)02276-5.
44. Grob CS. Deconstructing ecstasy: the politics of MDMA research. Addict Res. 2000;8(6):549–88.
45. Rogers G, Elston J, Garside R, Roome C, Taylor RS, Younger P, Somerville M. The harmful health effects of recreational ecstasy: a systematic review of observational evidence. Health Technol Assess. 2009;13 https://doi.org/10.3310/hta13050.
46. Morgan CJ, Curran HV, Independent Scientific Committee on Drugs. Ketamine use: a review. Addiction. 2012;107(1):27–38. https://doi.org/10.1111/j.1360-0443.2011.03576.x.
47. Wong GL-H, Tam Y-H, Ng C-F, Chan AW-H, Choi PC-L, Chu WC-W, Lai PB-S, Chan HL-Y, Wong VW-S. Liver injury is common among chronic abusers of ketamine. Clin Gastroenterol Hepatol. 2014;12(10):1759–1762.e1. https://doi.org/10.1016/j.cgh.2014.01.041.
48. Morgan CJ, Muetzelfeldt L, Curran HV. Consequences of chronic ketamine self-administration upon neurocognitive function and psychological wellbeing: a 1-year longitudinal study. Addiction. 2010;105(1):121–33. https://doi.org/10.1111/j.1360-0443.2009.02761.x.

# Inhalant Use Disorders

# 6

Rosemary Busch Conn

## Introduction

Though a less common substance use disorder, the unique features of inhalant use disorder create significant potential for severe morbidity and mortality. As defined by the DSM 5, inhalant use disorder is a problematic pattern of use of a hydrocarbon-based inhalant substance leading to clinically significant impairment or distress, as manifested by at least two of the ten criteria listed in Table 6.1 and occurring in a 12-month period [1].

Unique among its class and adding to its inconspicuous nature, inhalant use disorder has no corresponding withdrawal disorder. The differential diagnosis for inhalant use disorder includes unintentional inhalant exposure from industrial or other accidents; intentional inhalant use or intoxication that does not meet criteria for inhalant use disorder; inhalant-induced disorders (such as psychotic or depressive disorders); other substance use disorders, especially those involving sedating substances; other toxic, metabolic, traumatic, neoplastic, or infectious disorders impairing central or peripheral nervous system function; and disorders of other organ systems. Included among this class of substances are volatile solvents, aerosols, gases, and nitrites [1].

This chapter includes background information and epidemiology, two clinical cases on the topic at hand, physiologic consequences, and ends with treatment and prevention measures. Distinct features of this disorder include the multitude of substances which it encompasses and the variation of usage by population. The volume of specific substances in the category of inhalants results in difficulty classifying specific traits of this disorder and contributes to limited understanding of pharmacologic effects.

R. B. Conn (✉)
Adult Psychiatry Resident, New York Presbyterian – Weill Cornell Medicine,
New York, NY, USA
e-mail: Rvb9002@nyp.org



J. D. Avery, D. Hankins (eds.), *Addiction Medicine*, Psychiatry Update 2,
https://doi.org/10.1007/978-3-030-86430-9_6

**Table 6.1** Criteria of inhalant use disorder from DSM-5

| |
|---|
| Inhalant Use Disorder: a problematic pattern of use of a hydrocarbon-based inhalant substance leading to clinically significant impairment or distress |
| Occurs within a 12-month period |
| Includes at least two of the following criteria: |
| 1. The inhalant substance is often taken in larger amounts or over a longer period than was intended. |
| 2. There is a persistent desire or unsuccessful efforts to cut down or control use of the inhalant substance. |
| 3. A great deal of time is spent in activities necessary to obtain the inhalant substance, use it, or recover from its effects. |
| 4. Craving, or a strong desire or urge to use the inhalant substance. |
| 5. Recurrent use of the inhalant substance resulting in a failure to fulfill major role obligations at work, school, or home. |
| 6. Continued use of the inhalant substance despite having persistent or recurrent social or interpersonal problems caused or exacerbated by the effects of its use. |
| 7. Important social, occupational, or recreational activities are given up or reduced because of use of the inhalant substance. |
| 8. Recurrent use of the inhalant substance in situations in which it is physically hazardous. |
| 9. Use of the inhalant substance is continued despite knowledge of having a persistent or recurrent physical or psychological problem that is likely to have been caused or exacerbated by the substance. |
| 10. Tolerance, as defined by either of the following: |
| (a) A need for markedly increased amounts of the inhalant substance to achieve intoxication or desired effect |
| (b) A markedly diminished effect with continued use of the same amount of the inhalant substance |

## Epidemiology

There is some difficulty in establishing who meets criteria for inhalant use disorder, which is among the least prevalent substance use disorders. Broadly, inhalant use is most common among adolescents, with younger girls initially more likely to use than younger boys. This pattern eventually reverses with age, and young men are more likely to use inhalants than young women. Inhalant use occurs with higher prevalence in rural areas [2, 3].

According to the 2019 National Survey on Drug Use and Health, 807,000 people age 12 or older used inhalants in the prior month. That number increased to 2.1 million people (0.8% of the population) when the time frame was extended to a year, more than methamphetamine (2.0 million) and heroin (745,000). Estimates of the past year use increased since 2016 for people age 12 or above, with the primary shift seen in those aged 12–17 (from 2.2 percent in 2016 to 3.0 percent in 2019). Rates of use in young adults (ages 18–25) and adults above age 26 remained stable from 2015 to 2019. Of the 730,000 individuals who initiated inhalant use in 2019, slightly more than half were adolescents aged 12–17 (381,000) with an average of 1,000 adolescents initiating use each day. Across age groups, the number diagnosed with inhalant use disorder has remained stable at 0.4% since 2017 with adolescents constituting the highest proportion (0.3%) [4].

According to the national Youth Risk Behavior Survey (YRBS) published by the Centers for Disease Control and Prevention, the percentage of teens in grades 9–12 who have ever used inhalants– which is defined as having sniffed glue, breathed the contents of aerosol spray cans, or inhaled any paints or sprays to get high one or more times during their life– has decreased since 1995 (earliest data available). The percentage of lifetime use was 6.4% in 2019 [5].

## Case 1

Helen is a 14-year-old female with no significant medical history. She is preparing to begin 9th grade and lives in a rural part of her home state with her grandmother, who works as a cashier at the local grocery store, and two younger siblings. Both of Helen's parents have unknown substance use disorders. Her grandfather had bipolar I disorder and died 20 years prior from suicide.

Helen presents to her pediatrician, Dr. Chen, for her pre-high school physical exam. Before walking into the exam room where Helen and her grandmother are waiting, Dr. Chen looks over Helen's intake assessment. He immediately notices Helen's weight has dropped from the 40th percentile last year to below the 5th percentile. Her height has remained in the 50th percentile. Dr. Chen makes a note to evaluate for an eating disorder, as well as two things he sees more often than he would like in his rural pediatric practice: inadequate access to nutritious food and substance misuse.

Dr. Chen, Helen, and her grandmother discuss how things have been going since they met last winter when Helen was sick with a cold. He is relieved to know the grandmother is still working at the grocery store, where he knows she receives a discount on food. Helen describes that she spent the summer, "hanging out with my friends," and shrugs when pressed for details about how they were spending their time. Dr. Chen examines Helen, noticing as he checks her oropharynx that there are small erythematous papules on the skin surrounding her mouth. The remainder of Helen's exam is normal.

Dr. Chen tells Helen and her grandmother that he would like to speak with Helen individually. Helen opens up a little more and tells him that it has been difficult to have both of her parents away. Helen is open about having tried smoking a cigarette but did not like that it made her cough. She denies alcohol or cannabis use. When asked about other substances, she looks down and states that she started "bagging." Helen reports some friends were sniffing glue six months ago, since then she has been inhaling fumes, mostly from spray paint, out of a paper bag at least once a day. Dr. Chen asks Helen if she would be okay discussing this with her grandmother present. Helen is hesitant but agrees.

With Helen and her grandmother, Dr. Chen discusses the dangerous nature of using inhalants, answers their questions about it, and provides information about peer support groups for teenagers. Additionally, Dr. Chen makes a referral for Helen to see the child and adolescent psychiatrist in the closest nearby city, about half an hour from their rural town. He explains the importance of seeing the psychiatrist for additional help with inhalant use management and for psychiatric screening, especially with Helen's family history. When ordering lab tests, Dr. Chen includes urine hippuric acid and benzylmercapturic acid tests as well as a broad urine toxicology screen [2, 6, 7].

## Case 2

Benny is a 33-year-old gay male who works as a high school chemistry teacher. His medical history includes asthma and alcohol use disorder, which has been in remission since age 27. Following graduate school, Benny's alcohol use increased to the point that he was drinking every day and found he was unable to go without alcohol ingestion for more than a few days. But it was only after narrowly avoiding a car accident while driving intoxicated that he realized he needed to get professional help to stop using alcohol. Benny met with an addiction specialist who offered him a 30-day detoxification and rehabilitation program, as well as monthly injections of intramuscular naltrexone (Vivitrol). With an active Alcoholics Anonymous program and this medication, Benny has been able to refrain from using alcohol for over 5 years.

Benny lives in a large city with his dog. His family history includes alcohol use disorder in his father and grandfather. When his long-term relationship abruptly ended last year, Benny started attending parties with some younger friends to "blow off steam." At these parties he was introduced to "poppers." In addition to making him feel euphoric, the poppers were an enhancement to his sexual encounters.

Since the effects of poppers lasted only several minutes, Benny found that he was not impaired by them like he had been with alcohol. After attending a few parties where he used them, he learned the ease of buying them himself. His usage increased from occasional social use, to then using at home alone, and then bringing them to work. Inconspicuous and with a lingering odor indistinguishable from others in his chemistry laboratory classroom, Benny regularly used poppers at work between classes or on his lunch break.

This occurred for several weeks, until one Tuesday afternoon when Benny woke up confused in an ambulance. Another teacher found him unconscious and immediately called 911. In the emergency department, the EMS worker informed Dr. Willis that Benny was found holding a small canister of "liquid gold." He complained of a headache and gave inappropriate answers to orientation questions. On exam, he was tachycardic with a heart rate in the 140's and hypoxic with an oxygen saturation of 88% on room air. When nurse Chris drew his blood, he noticed how dark it appeared and informed Dr. Willis of this anomaly. Dr. Willis requested a nitrate test and a hemolysis panel in addition to basic lab tests. Due to a high index of suspicion for methemoglobinemia, she treated Benny with supplemental oxygen and IV methylene blue.

After recovery, Dr. Willis helped Benny call his addiction specialist and schedule an appointment for the following day [6, 8].

## Inhalant Classification, Psychosocial Impacts, Physiologic Effects, and Proposed Mechanisms

As a result of the wide range of products which vaporize, there were more than 200 different categories of inhalants reported between 1993 and 2008. To organize and classify the variety of inhalants, Storck et al. grouped them by chemical properties. In Group I are aliphatic, aromatic, or halogenated hydrocarbons, including propellants. Examples are fuels, such as toluene and gasoline, and computer sprays, which have seen a substantial increase in use since the early 2000s. Group II includes gases and other aerosols such as nitrous oxide, found in whipped cream dispensers and referred to colloquially as "whippets." Least used are inhalants in Group III which are the alkyl nitrates such as chlorohexyl nitrite [6].

The psychosocial impacts of inhalant use disorder are numerous though little is known about the natural history of inhalant use disorders and comorbidities in the general population. A common thread through the cases above is the association of inhalant use disorder with psychiatric conditions and, as in the second case, with other substance use disorders. Psychiatric conditions and symptoms notably more common among inhalant users include depressive disorders, anxiety disorders, suicidal ideation, and suicide attempts. Rates of depression and anxiety were higher in groups studied with occupational exposure to inhaled hydrocarbons. Though evident, differentiating whether this association is due to a similar spectrum of risk factors or if one is premorbid to the other is unclear. One hypothesis remarks on inhalant use as a global vulnerability marker, rather than a direct precipitant of psychiatric illness [6].

As there are many types of inhalants, the mechanism of use as well as signs and symptoms of intoxication or recent use can vary. The most common methods by which a vapor is inhaled are through direct inhalation from a container, inhalation from a product vaporized into a bag, or inhalation of fumes from a soaked cloth that covers the nose and/or mouth [8]. Signs of use can directly correlate to the method of ingestion. In the case of Helen, a perioral rash was evidence of recent use by inhaling fumes out of a paper bag, also known as "bagging."

Physiologic effects of inhalants correlate specifically to the substance ingested and broadly affect every organ system. Systems impacted are neurocognitive, metabolic, hepatic, renal, cardiovascular, hematopoietic, neuromuscular (including peripheral nerves), and reproductive. It is difficult to distinguish acute effects from those that result from sustained use as there have been reports of long-term impacts, such as in memory and processing speed, from a single occupational exposure. Occupational exposure studies allowed for the discovery of the effects of these substances on the body; however, these data serve only as a model due to higher exposure level in intentional inhalant use (whether by quantity, duration, or repetitious use) [6].

Acute physiologic effects mimic those of alcohol intoxication, such as dizziness, dysarthria, tremor, vision changes and involuntary eye movement, stupor, and coma, as well as impairments in cognition, coordination, and reflexes. With repetitive use, these temporary consequences progress to the development of encephalopathy, parkinsonism, cerebral atrophy, ataxia, and decreased cerebral perfusion. On brain imaging, hypointensities are visible in the thalamus and basal ganglia. Pulmonary dysfunction and disease are also highly common, with associations noted between duration of inhalant use and development of bronchitis, asthma, sinusitis, and tuberculosis. One study demonstrated an accelerated rate of radioisotope pulmonary clearance in those who were using inhaled solvents, indicating dysfunction at the level of the alveolar capillary membrane [6]. A particular example of physiologic impact relates to Benny from Case 2, which is that of amyl nitrate and its potential to cause methemoglobinemia; this can be fatal without recognition and timely treatment [8].

Additional adverse consequences of inhalant use are chemical and thermal burns, persistent mental illness, and medical emergencies. Severe and imminent life-threatening consequences of inhalant use are sudden sniffing death, asphyxiation, and unintentional injuries. Sudden sniffing death refers to heart failure precipitated by fatal arrhythmia [2, 6].

Cognitive and neurological effects can be temporary though with repeated exposure compounded deficits can be long-lasting. Global brain atrophy, as seen in Image B in Fig. 6.1, can occur in those with chronic toluene use [9]. Other effects of prolonged toluene exposure include impaired growth such that a person with

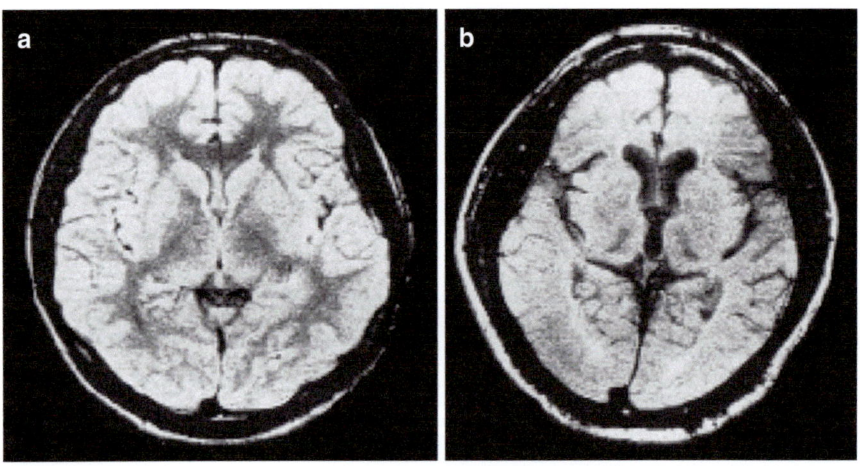


**Fig. 6.1** Normal brain (**a**) and brain with chronic exposure to inhalant (**b**). (Image **a** features the brain of a patient with no history of inhalant use. Image **b** features the brain of an individual who chronically uses toluene. The brain in image **b** has atrophied, evidenced by the smaller appearance and increased space inside the skull (the white outer circle in each image). *This image is used with permission from NIDA, Courtesy of Neil Rosenberg, M.D., NIDA Research Report (NIH 05-3818)* [9])

repeated use can develop failure to thrive, such as Helen in Case 1 [10]. Systemically, toluene inhalation can cause imminently harmful problems such as lactic acidosis, rhabdomyolysis, and acute hepatorenal injury [11].

Teratogenic effects occur with intrauterine exposure to inhaled substances. The presentation is similar to fetal alcohol syndrome with prominent features of facial and cranial deformities, poor brain development, low birth weight, developmental delays, as well as a variety of additional complications [4, 6].

The proposed mechanism for the neurobiology of inhalant use again varies by substance. Toluene and trichloroethylene promote motor excitation at low concentrations, whereas at high concentrations they potentiate anesthesia, sedation, coma, and even death. A proposed mechanism for toluene is that it blocks NMDA receptors in a similar way to PCP [4]. In studies with rats, toluene exposure increased dopamine levels in the prefrontal cortex and striatum, leading to increased neuron firing in the ventral tegmental area. This mechanism is similar to other substances which are misused. Benzene and diethyl ether work as depressants to the central nervous system as positive modulators to GABA-a receptors [4].

## Treatment

Treatment options for inhalant use disorder are limited; psychosocial treatments have shown some efficacy and pharmacologic options are minimal. Inadequate initiatives to develop treatment options can be attributed to lack of research, inadequate screening, and underreporting of use [4]. As with the case of Dr. Chen and Helen, directly approaching the patient is the foundation of treatment of inhalant use disorder. This method begins with the implementation of screening at every opportunity as well as looking out for signs of use, such as Helen's perioral dermatitis and failure to thrive. The SBIRT model offers a standardized approach to screening and intervention that includes questions on topics of frequency and amount of use, as well as impacts of use on personal and interpersonal functioning [12]. As with other substance use disorders, the motivational interview is crucial in determining the state of readiness of change for a particular patient, as well as guiding them along in the process [13]. Outpatient and inpatient substance use treatment programs, which utilize structured environments, peer support, individual and group counseling, education, and accountability, can be useful in the treatment of inhalant use disorder [4].

Primary prevention methods aim to deter the use of commonly used volatile compounds and are a key area of focus in reducing harm from inhalant abuse [4]. Examples of primary prevention include clearer labeling for misused products and chemicals, changing the composition of products so the volatile chemicals causing intoxication are replaced or masked, monitoring quantity of particular products purchased, and the addition of age restrictions. Other harm reduction strategies are to make usage safer, such as advising persons to avoid the use of compounds containing propane and butane, refrain from placing a plastic bag over one's head, and take precautions to avoid burns, overdose, and aspiration of vomitus.

Treatment at the community level is multipart. Nearly every rural community needs increased access to mental health care and substance use treatment. Educational initiatives and outreach programs directly addressing substance use are imperative in prevention of all substance use disorders, including inhalants. Opportunities for youth engagement such as recreational programs offer a means of alternative time spent for youth most vulnerable to early substance use. Culturally sensitive outreach and education may be critical in certain vulnerable communities. In Canada and Australia, for example, holistic approaches that utilize components drawn from indigenous cultures have been shown to be efficacious treatment options for inhalant use disorder in indigenous populations [4].

Pharmacological treatments for inhalant use disorder have not been well researched, though some antipsychotics and antiepileptic agents demonstrate benefit for symptom relief. In one case report of a patient who developed psychotic symptoms after repeated gasoline inhalation, the administration of risperidone led to both decreased psychotic symptoms and decreased cravings. Haloperidol and carbamazepine similarly have some limited evidence for decreasing symptoms in those with inhalant-induced psychotic disorders. A case report showed reduction in cravings and increased abstinence with lamotrigine [4].

## Conclusion

Although inhalant use disorder is relatively rare compared to other substance use disorders, it can nevertheless cause significant injury to those affected by it, including several potentially fatal complications. Inhalant use should be part of any comprehensive substance use screening, particularly when working with populations with higher prevalence of the disorder. Although treatment options are limited, some of the psychosocial treatments with efficacy in other substance use disorders have also been shown to work in this patient population.

### Key Points

- Inhalant use disorder describes problematic use of a heterogeneous group of substances including volatile solvents, aerosols, gases, and nitrites.
- Inhalants can exert their effects across body systems both acutely (including life-threatening hematologic, respiratory, and cardiac risks) and more chronically.
- Careful screening, harm reduction, and community-level interventions are critical to reducing the burden of disease.
- Treatment options for inhalant use are primarily psychosocial and overlap with those for other substance use disorders.

## References


1. Kalai. Diagnostic and statistical manual of mental disorders: DSM-5. Arlington: American Psychiatric Association; 2017. p. 533–40.
2. Storck M, Black L, Liddell M. Inhalant abuse and dextromethorphan. Child Adolesc Psychiatr Clin N Am. 2016;25:497–508.
3. Crossin R, Scott D, Witt KG, Duncan JR, Smith K, Lubman DI. Acute harms associated with inhalant misuse: co-morbidities and trends relative to age and gender among ambulance attendees. Drug Alcohol Depend. 2018;190:46–53.
4. National Institute on Drug Abuse. Inhalants trends & statistics. National Institute on Drug Abuse; 2020. https://www.drugabuse.gov/drug-topics/inhalants/inhalants-trends-statistics. Accessed 15 Feb 2021.
5. Kalai. Trends in the prevalence of marijuana, cocaine, and other illegal drug use national YRBS: 1991–2019. Centers for Disease Control and Prevention; 2020. https://www.cdc.gov/healthyyouth/data/yrbs/factsheets/2019_us_drug_trend_yrbs.htm
6. Howard MO, Bowen SE, Garland EL, Perron BE, Vaughn MG. Inhalant use and inhalant use disorders in the United States. Addiction Science & Clinical Practice; 2011. https://www.ncbi.nlm.nih.gov/pmc/articles/PMC3188822/
7. Crossin R, Cairney S, Lawrence AJ, Duncan JR. Adolescent inhalant abuse leads to other drug use and impaired growth; implications for diagnosis. Aust N Z J Public Health. 2016;41:99–104.
8. Hunter L, Gordge L, Dargan PI, Wood DM. Methaemoglobinaemia associated with the use of cocaine and volatile nitrites as recreational drugs: a review. Br J Clin Pharmacol. 2011;72:18–26.
9. National Institute on Drug Abuse. What are the other medical consequences of inhalant abuse? National Institute on Drug Abuse; 2020. https://www.drugabuse.gov/publications/research-reports/inhalants/what-are-other-medical-consequences-inhalant-abuse
10. Crossin R, Qama A, Andrews ZB, Lawrence AJ, Duncan JR. The effect of adolescent inhalant abuse on energy balance and growth. Pharmacol Res Perspect. 2019;7(4):e00498. https://doi.org/10.1002/prp2.498.
11. Camara-Lemarroy CR, Rodríguez-Gutiérrez R, Monreal-Robles R, González-González JG. Acute toluene intoxication–clinical presentation, management and prognosis: a prospective observational study. BMC Emerg Med. 2015;15:19. https://www.ncbi.nlm.nih.gov/pmc/articles/PMC4539858/
12. Tools. Clinician tools – SBIRT for substance abuse. https://www.sbirt.care/tools.aspx. Accessed 15 Feb 2021.
13. Empowering change: motivational interviewing. SAMHSA. https://www.samhsa.gov/homelessness-programs-resources/hpr-resources/empowering-change. Accessed 15 Feb 2021.

# Opioid Use Disorder

# 7

Sierra Ferguson and Aviva Teitelbaum

## Introduction

Opioid use disorder is defined by the chronic use of opioids that leads to clinically significant impairment or distress [1]. Opioid use disorder is diagnosed when an individual meets two or more of the 11 criteria in the table below within a one-year period, and severity is based on the number of symptoms present (Table 7.1). An estimated 26.8 million people globally have opioid use disorder with over 100,000 overdose deaths reported each year [2]. In 2018, 10.3 million people or 3.7% of the US population aged 12 or older were estimated to have misused opioids, and two million of these individuals met criteria for opioid use disorder [3]. An estimated 446,000 American died from an opioid overdose from 1999 to 2018 and of those 233,000 died from a prescription opioid overdose [4]. During this same time period, there was a tenfold increase in overdose deaths caused by fentanyl [4], a synthetic opioid 30–50 times more potent than heroin [5, 6]. The prevalence of heroin use in the United States has increased significantly over the past two decades, doubling in number from 2002 to 2018 [7], and two thirds of individuals who use heroin also report use of prescription opioids [8]. Given the increasing rates of opioid overdose deaths and the human toll caused by this "opioid epidemic," in 2017, the US Department of Health and Human Services declared the opioid crisis a public health emergency, which increased public funding for treatment, overdose prevention, and training of first responders and other medical professionals to respond to the crisis [9].

S. Ferguson
Icahn School of Medicine at Mount Sinai, Mount Sinai Health System, New York, NY, USA
e-mail: Sierra.Ferguson@mountsinai.org

A. Teitelbaum (✉)
NYU Grossman School of Medicine, New York, NY, USA
e-mail: Aviva.Teitelbaum@nyulangone.org



J. D. Avery, D. Hankins (eds.), *Addiction Medicine*, Psychiatry Update 2,
https://doi.org/10.1007/978-3-030-86430-9_7

**Table 7.1** DSM-5 diagnostic criteria for opioid use disorder [1]

| |
|---|
| Opioids are often taken in larger amounts or over a longer period of time than intended |
| There is a persistent desire or unsuccessful efforts to cut down or control opioid use |
| A great deal of time is spent in activities necessary to obtain the opioid, use the opioid, or recover from its effects |
| Craving, or a strong desire to use opioids |
| Recurrent opioid use resulting in failure to fulfill major role obligations at work, school, or home |
| Continued opioid use despite having persistent or recurrent social or interpersonal problems caused or exacerbated by the effects of opioids |
| Important social, occupational, or recreational activities are given up or reduced because of opioid use |
| Recurrent opioid use in situations in which it is physically hazardous |
| Continued use despite knowledge of having a persistent or recurrent physical or psychological problem that is likely to have been caused or exacerbated by opioids |
| Tolerance, as defined by either of the following: (a) a need for markedly increased amounts of opioids to achieve intoxication or desired effect or (b) a markedly diminished effect with continued use of the same amount of an opioid |
| Withdrawal, as manifested by either of the following: (a) the characteristic opioid withdrawal syndrome or (b) the same (or a closely related) substance is taken to relieve or avoid withdrawal symptoms |

Individuals develop opioid use disorder through a variety of pathways including legitimate use or abuse of prescription analgesics such as oxycodone and hydrocodone or through use of illicit substances such as heroin. Individuals at risk for developing opioid use disorder frequently have risk factors including current or past history of substance abuse, introduction to opioids at a younger age, untreated psychiatric disorders, and social and familial contexts where substance use is commonplace [10].

Medication-assisted treatment for opioid use disorder, when used in conjunction with psychosocial interventions and counseling, shows superior treatment outcomes in terms of treatment retention, lower mortality, and improved quality of life [11–14]. Despite strong evidence in support of MAT, it is underutilized [15, 16]. This can be explained in part due to stigma held by both patients and providers, lack of training for providers particularly in rural areas, and limited access to opioid treatment programs [17, 18]. One study found that less than 50% of privately funded substance use disorder treatment programs offer MAT as part of their treatment programs and of those only 34.4% of patients with opioid use disorder received MAT [19]. The goal of this chapter is to illustrate the evolution of an opioid use disorder (OUD) through a clinical case and to outline the pharmacologic treatment options to treat this illness including methadone, an opioid agonist; buprenorphine, an opioid partial agonist; and naltrexone, an opioid antagonist.

## Clinical Case

Joe is a 45-year-old married man, working in construction, who sustained a work-related injury; while using a circular saw to cut a piece of wood, he accidentally sliced off his index finger. Fortunately, he salvaged his finger, and it was reattached at a nearby hospital. Dr. Frank, the surgeon who performed the procedure, prescribed Joe a one-month supply of oxycodone-acetaminophen (commonly known as Percocet) to treat his postoperative pain.

Prior to receiving this prescription for oxycodone-acetaminophen, Joe had never used any opioid analgesics nor any illicit opioids. He considered himself a "social drinker," but never drank on a daily basis, infrequently got drunk, and never blacked out from alcohol. His wife, however, did have a remote history of heroin addiction and was on methadone prescribed by an opioid treatment program (OTP) in a nearby town. Joe did not have any chronic medical conditions, nor did he have any relevant psychiatric history. He recalls his father being "an angry drunk," but his parents divorced at a young age, and he never maintained a relationship with his father after he left.

Joe began taking the opioid analgesic as his doctor had prescribed it. Initially, the medication adequately controlled Joe's pain, but within a few weeks, the pain in his finger became more intense. In an attempt to help alleviate Joe's pain, Dr. Frank renewed Joe's prescription and doubled his supply during the following 2 months.

Four months after Joe's procedure, despite ongoing complaints of intense "dagger-like" pain in his reattached index finger, Dr. Frank informed Joe that he could no longer continue to prescribe oxycodone-acetaminophen, explaining "the medical community is cracking down on narcotic prescriptions, so you should try to cope without the medication." At this point, Joe had been consuming oxycodone-acetaminophen 5–325 mg up to six times daily for several months. He was worried about being suddenly cut off from his prescription, recalling a time when he had forgotten his pain medication at home during a work day, and he experienced flu-like symptoms of opioid withdrawal. He expressed these concerns to his doctor who offered to refer him to a pain management specialist, but the next available appointment was in 3 months' time.

In the week following his last appointment with Dr. Frank, Joe attempted to cut back on his oxycodone-acetaminophen use. He had about 30 pills remaining, and he attempted to reduce his use from six pills daily to three pills daily. He succeeded at this, despite enduring numerous symptoms of opioid withdrawal: chills, muscle aches, nausea, and diarrhea. Joe felt like he had come down with a terrible bout of influenza. His wife, concerned about his state, suggested he enroll at her opioid treatment program and initiate methadone. Joe refused. He had always regarded methadone as "legal heroin" and had been encouraging his wife to taper off of it.

As he only had a few days' supply of pain medications remaining, and his pain management appointment was still ten weeks away, Joe felt that he had to find an interim solution. He took to the Internet to search his options, and he found a compound called kratom (*Mitragyna speciosa*), which could be bought legally, marketed itself as an effective painkiller, and had opioid-like properties that would soften the impact of opioid withdrawal.

Joe found relief in kratom – a powder he brewed into hot water – which he consumed multiple times daily. It lessened his symptoms of opioid withdrawal and dulled the pain in his finger. He noticed, however, that he quickly became tolerant of kratom. He began by drinking three cups of kratom daily, and within a few weeks, he was drinking six cups daily to achieve the same desired effect.

Joe started to worry about the financial implications of his new kratom habit. His wife approached him again and suggested that he come to her Opioid Treatment Program and hear about the available treatment options, assuring him that methadone is not the only option for his condition. Joe agreed.

## Pharmacologic Interventions

When Joe arrives at the clinic, he meets with a psychiatrist to discuss treatment options and shares that he last used kratom yesterday morning and is already experiencing withdrawal symptoms and cravings to use again. During the visit a Clinical Opiate Withdrawal Scale (COWS) is administered, which is an 11-item scale designed to assess withdrawal symptoms over time, rating withdrawal symptoms from mild, moderate, moderately severe, and severe [20]. Joe's vitals are taken and blood pressure is 125/90 mm Hg and pulse rate 110 beats per minute. He blows his nose several times as he enters the exam room and reports feeling anxious and restless with strong urges to use kratom. He is noted to be sweating and yawns twice during the session. He also reports experiencing severe muscle and bone pain and gets up several times during the interview to use the bathroom due to nausea and severe diarrhea. Based on these symptoms of opioid withdrawal, Joe's COWS score is 16, indicating moderate withdrawal. He is not noted to have any tremor or gooseflesh skin, and pupils appear normal-sized. Joe initially states he wants to "tough it out" and detox from kratom without MAT due to concern for "getting addicted to something else." Detox options are discussed, specifically non-opioid symptomatic treatment of opioid withdrawal including clonidine 0.1–0.2 mg four times daily to treat Joe's tachycardia, anxiety, sweating, and hypertension. Metoclopramide 10 mg every 6 hours as needed is offered for nausea and loperamide 4 mg initially, and then 2 mg thereafter (up to 16 mg/day) is offered for diarrhea. Ibuprofen 400 mg three times daily as needed is offered for pain, and he is also prescribed trazodone 50 mg nightly as needed for insomnia which he also reported experiencing due to the withdrawal [21].

By the end of the 45-minute session, Joe appeared even more restless and was noted to have a new onset tremor and a COWS score of 23. As he rose to leave the

**Table 7.2** Pros and cons of the three FDA-approved treatments for OUD

| Medication | Pros | Cons |
|---|---|---|
| Methadone | Medication cost is affordable [50]<br>Straightforward induction process<br>Reduction in infectious disease transmission and criminal activity [51]<br>Safely used in pregnancy [52]<br>Some find benefit to the structure of an OTP<br>Low risk of diversion due to strict initial frequent attendance policy | Initially 6 day/week attendance expected at most OTPs<br>No office-based treatment, must have access to OTP [24]<br>Cardiac arrhythmias [53]<br>Overdose risk [24]<br>Stigmatized<br>High abuse potential<br>At high doses: sedation, constipation, sexual dysfunction [54] |
| Buprenorphine | Ceiling effect: low risk of overdose, less abuse potential<br>Daily or alternate-day dosing<br>Increased flexibility: office-based prescribing<br>Less stigmatized than methadone<br>Safely used in pregnancy [55] | Costly: medication is moderately expensive, and DEA-X waivered physicians usually in private practice<br>Moderate abuse potential [55]<br>Diversion risk with office-based prescribing<br>Risk of precipitated withdrawal during induction [55] |
| Naltrexone | Blocks high from any opioid use<br>Relieves cravings<br>No risk of naltrexone withdrawal<br>Less stigmatized than methadone<br>Minimal abuse potential | Risk of precipitated withdrawal during induction<br>Decreases tolerance, therefore increases overdose risk<br>Common side effect: nausea |

office, he walked to the door then stopped and turned around and said "I'd actually like to hear about the other treatment options. I can't continue withdrawing like this."

The psychiatrist welcomed Joe back into the room and provided supportive listening about how much Joe has struggled with his chronic pain and resultant opioid dependence. She then reviewed the three FDA-approved medication options for opioid use disorder that work by reducing cravings: methadone, buprenorphine, and naltrexone [22].

The psychiatrist, aware that Joe's wife was treated with methadone for opioid use disorder, began by discussing this option. Methadone, she explained, is a long-acting opioid agonist that is FDA-approved for both opioid use disorder and pain management, which could be helpful for Joe's finger pain [23]. She also shared that methadone can only be dispensed by a SAMHSA-certified Opioid Treatment Program (OTP) that would provide on-site administration of methadone in liquid form six days a week along with individual sessions with a counselor, regular urine toxicology, and group therapy. Additional pros and cons of methadone were reviewed with Joe (Table 7.2) [24].

Joe expressed interest in the pain management aspects of methadone though expressed hesitance that methadone was not for him, saying "it seems like yet another drug to abuse."

Next the psychiatrist reviewed naltrexone, a synthetic opioid antagonist, as a treatment option given that there is no abuse potential with this medication [25]. She explained how this medication was available as a tablet or in an extended-release monthly injection called Vivitrol that could be prescribed in an outpatient clinic setting. Naltrexone functions by binding to and blocking the opioid receptor [25] and by extension would block opioid-like substances such as kratom, which has agonist effects on the opioid receptor. Naltrexone therefore reduces opioid cravings and compulsive opioid use [3]. Joe seemed interested initially, though when he learned that he would have to remain abstinent from opioids or opioid-like substances for 6 days prior to induction on naltrexone, he declined this option.

Aware that Joe was seeking a more immediate treatment for his opioid cravings and withdrawal, the psychiatrist then recommended buprenorphine, an opioid partial agonist that can be prescribed in an outpatient clinic setting. Given Joe's current withdrawal symptoms, he could safely be induced on buprenorphine today in the office. The treatment, it was explained, would reduce his opioid cravings and withdrawal symptoms as well as reduce some of his finger pain given its action at the opioid receptor. The pros and cons of this treatment were reviewed with Joe including risk for precipitated withdrawal – if he had recently consumed opioids – and potential side effects. Various formulation options were reviewed including buprenorphine sublingual tablets (Subutex), buprenorphine-naloxone combination sublingual films (Suboxone) and tablets (Zubsolv), as well as longer-acting forms of buprenorphine such as extended-release injection (Sublocade). Given Joe's concern about the abuse potential of his treatment, he opted to try a buprenorphine-naloxone compound, since naloxone reduces misuse of buprenorphine. Joe agreed to start buprenorphine-naloxone combination sublingual films (Suboxone) 4 mg in the office and would return home with an additional 4 mg to take that evening if withdrawal symptoms persisted. He agreed to return the following morning for assessment and potential dose adjustment. See treatment Algorithm 7.1 for additional guidance of initiating MAT for the treatment of opioid use disorder.

## Discussion

Joe's story is similar to that of many thousands of Americans who have developed an opioid use disorder over the past 30 years. In 1995, the American Pain Society (APS) set out guidelines that encouraged medical providers to record patients' reports of pain, with the goal of improving the diagnosis and treatment of pain. They recommended that patients' reports of pain should be taken as seriously as vital sign measurements, thereby coining this initiative *pain as the fifth vital sign* [32]. Not surprisingly, an increase in pain assessments brought on an increase in opioid analgesic prescribing; opioid prescriptions increased from 76 million in 1991 to 219 million in 2011. Unfortunately, during this time of widespread opioid prescribing, pharmaceutical companies marketed opioid analgesics to the medical community as non-addictive [33], which we now recognize is not the case. The increase in opioid prescriptions led to an increase in opioid-related emergency room visits, treatment admissions, and overdose fatalities [34].

In response to the increasing rates of controlled substance misuse in the United States, prescription drug monitoring programs (PDMPs) were implemented in most

American states. With the implementation of PDMPs, there was a corresponding 30 percent decrease in the rates of prescribing Schedule II opioids (which includes most prescription opioids) [35]. Physicians became increasingly aware of the addictive nature of prescription opioids, and many abruptly changed their prescribing practices, sometimes to the detriment of their patients.

Naloxone, a rapid-acting opioid receptor antagonist, was introduced to the market in a more user-friendly form in recent years. In the past, this medication had been used only in medical settings such as emergency rooms, since it was only available in intravenous or intramuscular form. Importantly, the key to reversing an opioid overdose is prompt timing of naloxone administration, so the recent creation and wider distribution of an easy-to-use intranasal naloxone spray have been an important step in overdose prevention [36]. Naloxone should be prescribed to anyone considered high risk of opioid overdose – such as individuals with an opioid use disorder who have recently been released from a period of incarceration or those who are prescribed high doses of long-acting opioid analgesics – and a doctor or pharmacist can show patients, their family members, or caregivers how to administer intranasal naloxone [37].

As was seen in Joe's case, his doctor abruptly stopped his opioid prescription, leaving Joe without access to a medication he was physiologically dependent on. It is at this juncture that many people make the transition to heroin due to its widespread availability, adequate analgesic effect, and affordability. In Joe's case, however, he harbored considerable stigma about illicit drugs and their treatments, such as methadone, so he sought out kratom, an opioid-like compound that is sold legally online and in head shops. Kratom (*Mitragyna speciosa*) is harvested from a tree indigenous to Southeast Asia and is a relative of the coffee plant. It is sold as a powder that can be stirred into a beverage or put in individual capsules for consumption. At lower doses, kratom has stimulant-like properties, and at higher doses it behaves like an opioid, and in fact is an agonist on the major opioid receptors. In recent years it has gained popularity as a recreational drug that is marketed to improve mood, relieve pain, and may provide benefit in opioid addiction [38]. As we saw in the above case, Joe became tolerant of kratom and began to use higher doses to achieve the same effect. Upon recognizing this, he agreed to visit his wife's OTP and consider a medication-assisted treatment for opioid use disorder.

Upon learning about the three FDA-approved treatments for opioid use disorder, Joe found himself most partial to buprenorphine-naloxone combination therapy (Suboxone). He told the psychiatrist that he heard that methadone causes dental and bone decay. The OTP psychiatrist explained that methadone can reduce the production of saliva, which prevents dental caries. Therefore, initiating methadone can cause dry mouth, which may increase risk of cavities; however, methadone does not directly act on the teeth to cause dental decay. Additionally, until arriving at a therapeutic dose of methadone, opioid withdrawal symptoms may cause musculoskeletal pain, which may be misconstrued as bone breakdown. Methadone does not directly act on bones to break them down, however. Joe mentioned that he is also worried that people would regard him as "weak and without willpower" if he agreed to methadone or another MAT [39]. His wife has been on methadone for nearly a decade, and he is worried that if he were to start it, he would never get off. While the OTP psychiatrist understood that there is considerable stigma against people with substance use disorders and those on MAT, she assured Joe that most providers he would be working with at the clinic would see his seeking treatment as a sign of willpower: he is asking for help with a habit that has become destructive. She also assured Joe that every patient is different: some patients use MAT as a bridge to transitioning off opioids altogether, and others need to be on MAT for many years, given how susceptible they are to relapse on opioids.

Despite the OTP psychiatrist debunking many of Joe's preconceived notions about methadone, and recommending it for the dual treatment of opioid use disorder and pain management, Joe opted to initiate suboxone. While he could initiate suboxone at his wife's OTP, he preferred to find an office-based suboxone provider in the future, so he would not be subject to the initial six-day-per-week pickup schedule of the OTP.

Despite substantial evidence for its efficacy, safety, and relative ease of use, buprenorphine remains vastly underutilized [40]. In order to become a licensed buprenorphine prescriber, one must provide MAT in a qualified practice setting or hold board certification in addiction medicine or addiction psychiatry. Buprenorphine training is typically eight hours in duration and grants those a DEA X waiver to prescribe buprenorphine [41]. As of 2017, more than half (56.3%) of US counties were without a buprenorphine prescriber [42]. In addition, most waivered physicians treat far fewer than the potential maximum of 275 patients they are eligible to treat. Studies suggest a lack of prescriber experience and education in the use of buprenorphine as a reason for its underutilization [43]. Buprenorphine has also been criticized as being marketed to a specifically white, affluent, college-educated population [44]. Notably its advertising campaigns do not target an underserved population with low socioeconomic status, where rates of substance use disorders are highest. In addition, many state-funded Medicaid programs do not cover reimbursements for buprenorphine, thereby narrowing the scope of prescribing to more affluent subsections of the population with private insurance [45].

## Psychotherapeutic and Psychosocial Interventions

The treatment of opioid use disorder includes medication-assisted treatment as well as a range of behavioral interventions aimed at helping patients to reduce urges to use opioids, maintain abstinence, and develop coping skills [46]. Studies have shown superior clinical outcomes in the treatment of opioid use disorder when medication management was combined with psychosocial interventions [47]. These interventions take the form of individual and group therapies including cognitive behavioral therapy, acceptance and commitment therapy, couples and family therapy including network therapy, contingency management, motivational interviewing, social skills training, harm reduction counseling, and 12-step facilitation therapy [48]. Some treatments such as 12-step facilitation therapy (such as Narcotics Anonymous, with almost 20,000 groups worldwide) promote an abstinence-only recovery approach, while others such as harm reduction counseling seek primarily to reduce the negative sequelae of substance use, such as infectious disease transmission or criminal behavior.

Joe's case provides a good example of where motivational interviewing could be used to help Joe recognize problems associated with his kratom use, explore and resolve ambivalence about his use, and explore both the benefits of changing his addictive behaviors and the costs of not changing. In this case, the OTP psychiatrist could take a nonjudgmental stance and use empathy to align with Joe in his struggle to stop using kratom. She could employ open-ended questioning and reflections to help Joe to see the gap between his kratom use and his personal goals and values. The psychiatrist could elicit Joe's own reasons for change referred to as "change talk" rather than trying to persuade him that he should stop using kratom. She could also explore his belief about MAT being a sign of weakness rather than as a sign of strength in his recovery.

## Conclusion

The opioid epidemic is one of the most profound public health crises that the United States has faced over the course of its history. An increase in opioid analgesic prescribing in the late 1990s and early 2000s led to an increase in misuse and abuse of prescription opioids, which commonly became a gateway to developing a heroin addiction [49]. There are three medication-assisted treatments [13] for opioid use disorder – methadone, buprenorphine, and naltrexone – and they are all underprescribed and heavily stigmatized, both by the lay public, by patients with opioid use disorders, and even by medical providers. This chapter has attempted to illustrate how a middle-aged man without a prior history of addiction developed an opioid use disorder through a legitimate prescription by his own physician. Within a short period of time, he was physiologically dependent on opioid analgesics and later on kratom, an opioid-like compound that reduces opioid withdrawal symptoms. The patient's own long-held beliefs about MAT prevented him from seeking treatment immediately and from weighing all three approved treatment options equally. While the psychiatrist in this case was well-versed on each approved MAT for the patient's opioid use disorder, MAT in general is vastly underprescribed, possibly due to prescriber lack of training and experience in MAT prescribing. Additional efforts in educating medical providers and the general public on the disease of addiction and its treatments are a necessary step in tackling the opioid epidemic.

## Algorithm 7.1 Treatment of Opioid Use Disorder

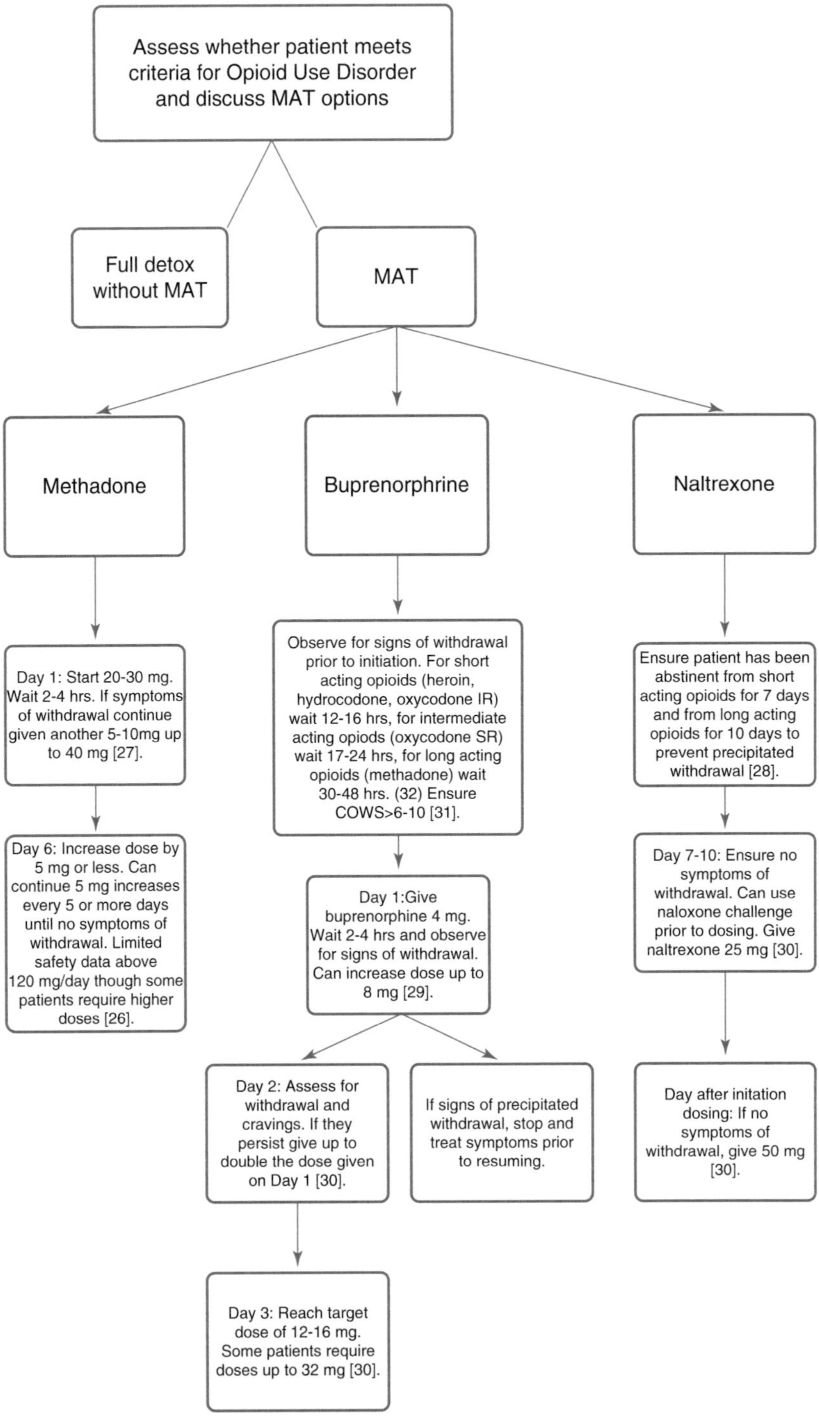

## References


1. American Psychiatric Association. Diagnostic criteria for opioid use disorder. Diagnostic and statistical manual of mental disorders. 5th ed. Arlington: APA; 2013.
2. GBD 2016 Disease and Injury Incidence and Prevalence Collaborators. Global, regional, and national incidence, prevalence, and years lived with disability for 328 diseases and injuries for 195 countries, 1990-2016: a systematic analysis for the Global Burden of Disease Study 2016. Lancet. 2017;390(10100):1211–59.
3. American Society of Addiction Medicine. National practice guideline for the treatment of opioid use disorder: 2020 focused update 2020. Available from: www.asam.org
4. Centers for Disease Control and Prevention, National Center for Health Statistics. Multiple causes of death 1999–2018. Wide-ranging online data for epidemiologic research (WONDER) Atlanta 2019. Available from: http://wonder.cdc.gov
5. Han Y, Yan W, Zheng Y, Khan MZ, Yuan K, Lu L. The rising crisis of illicit fentanyl use, overdose, and potential therapeutic strategies. Transl Psychiatry. 2019;9(1):282.
6. Poklis A. Fentanyl: a review for clinical and analytical toxicologists. J Toxicol Clin Toxicol. 1995;33(5):439–47.
7. Han B, Volkow ND, Compton WM, McCance-Katz EF. Reported heroin use, use disorder, and injection among adults in the United States, 2002–2018. JAMA. 2020;323(6):568–71.
8. Rosenblum A, Parrino M, Schnoll SH, Fong C, Maxwell C, Cleland CM, et al. Prescription opioid abuse among enrollees into methadone maintenance treatment. Drug Alcohol Depend. 2007;90(1):64–71.
9. Gostin LO, Hodge JG Jr, Noe SA. Reframing the opioid epidemic as a national emergency. JAMA. 2017;318(16):1539–40.
10. Webster LR. Risk factors for opioid-use disorder and overdose. Anesth Analg. 2017;125(5):1741–8.
11. Bell J, Strang J. Medication treatment of opioid use disorder. Biol Psychiatry. 2020;87(1):82–8.
12. Kelty E, Joyce D, Hulse G. A retrospective cohort study of mortality rates in patients with an opioid use disorder treated with implant naltrexone, oral methadone or sublingual buprenorphine. Am J Drug Alcohol Abuse. 2019;45(3):285–91.
13. Mattick RP, Breen C, Kimber J, Davoli M. Methadone maintenance therapy versus no opioid replacement therapy for opioid dependence. Cochrane Database Syst Rev. 2009;(3):CD002209.
14. Timko C, Schultz NR, Cucciare MA, Vittorio L, Garrison-Diehn C. Retention in medication-assisted treatment for opiate dependence: a systematic review. J Addict Dis. 2016;35(1):22–35.
15. Neighbors CJ, Choi S, Healy S, Yerneni R, Sun T, Shapoval L. Age related medication for addiction treatment (MAT) use for opioid use disorder among Medicaid-insured patients in New York. Subst Abuse Treat Prev Policy. 2019;14(1):28.
16. Robertson AG, Easter MM, Lin H, Frisman LK, Swanson JW, Swartz MS. Medication-assisted treatment for alcohol-dependent adults with serious mental illness and criminal justice involvement: effects on treatment utilization and outcomes. Am J Psychiatry. 2018;175(7):665–73.
17. Cicero TJ, Surratt H, Inciardi JA, Munoz A. Relationship between therapeutic use and abuse of opioid analgesics in rural, suburban, and urban locations in the United States. Pharmacoepidemiol Drug Saf. 2007;16(8):827–40.
18. Knudsen HK, Ducharme LJ, Roman PM. Research network involvement and addiction treatment center staff: counselor attitudes toward buprenorphine. Am J Addict. 2007;16(5):365–71.
19. Knudsen HK, Abraham AJ, Roman PM. Adoption and implementation of medications in addiction treatment programs. J Addict Med. 2011;5(1):21–7.
20. Wesson DR, Ling W. The clinical opiate withdrawal scale (COWS). J Psychoactive Drugs. 2003;35(2):253–9.
21. WHO. Clinical guidelines for withdrawal management and treatment of drug dependence in closed settings. Geneva: WHO; 2009. Available from: https://www.ncbi.nlm.nih.gov/books/NBK310654/

22. Bart G. Maintenance medication for opiate addiction: the foundation of recovery. J Addict Dis. 2012;31(3):207–25.
23. U.S. Food and Drug Administration. Methadone. Available from: https://www.fda.gov/media/76020/download
24. U.S. Department of Health and Human Services, Substance Abuse and Mental Health Services Administration, Methadone 2021. Available from: https://www.samhsa.gov/medication-assisted-treatment/medications-counseling-related-conditions/methadone
25. U.S. Department of Health and Human Services, Substance Abuse and Mental Health Services Administration, Naltrexone 2020. Available from: https://www.samhsa.gov/medication-assisted-treatment/medications-counseling-related-conditions/naltrexone
26. Baxter LE Sr, Campbell A, Deshields M, Levounis P, Martin JA, McNicholas L, et al. Safe methadone induction and stabilization: report of an expert panel. J Addict Med. 2013;7(6):377–86.
27. Joseph H, Stancliff S, Langrod J. Methadone maintenance treatment (MMT): a review of historical and clinical issues. Mt Sinai J Med. 2000;67(5–6):347–64.
28. O'Connor PG, Fiellin DA. Pharmacologic treatment of heroin-dependent patients. Ann Intern Med. 2000;133(1):40–54.
29. Johnson RE, Strain EC, Amass L. Buprenorphine: how to use it right. Drug Alcohol Depend. 2003;70(2 Suppl):S59–77.
30. U.S. Department of Health and Human Services, Substance Abuse and Mental Health Services Administration. Medication-assisted treatment for opioid addiction in opioid treatment programs. SAMHSA/CSAT treatment improvement protocols. Rockville: U.S. Department of Health and Human Services, Substance Abuse and Mental Health Services Administration; 2005.
31. Nielsen S, Hillhouse M, Weiss RD, Mooney L, Sharpe Potter J, Lee J, et al. The relationship between primary prescription opioid and buprenorphine-naloxone induction outcomes in a prescription opioid dependent sample. Am J Addict. 2014;23(4):343–8.
32. Quality improvement guidelines for the treatment of acute pain and cancer pain. American pain society quality of care committee. JAMA. 1995;274(23):1874–80.
33. U.S. Department of Health and Human Services. What is the U.S. opioid epidemic 2019. Available from: https://www.hhs.gov/opioids/about-the-epidemic/index.html
34. Cicero TJ, Ellis MS. The prescription opioid epidemic: a review of qualitative studies on the progression from initial use to abuse. Dialogues Clin Neurosci. 2017;19(3):259–69.
35. Bao Y, Pan Y, Taylor A, Radakrishnan S, Luo F, Pincus HA, et al. Prescription drug monitoring programs are associated with sustained reductions in opioid prescribing by physicians. Health Aff (Millwood). 2016;35(6):1045–51.
36. Lin LA, Brummett CM, Waljee JF, Englesbe MJ, Gunaseelan V, Bohnert ASB. Association of opioid overdose risk factors and naloxone prescribing in US adults. J Gen Intern Med. 2020;35(2):420–7.
37. U.S. Department of Health and Human Services, Substance Abuse and Mental Health Services Administration. Naloxone 2020. Available from: https://www.samhsa.gov/medication-assisted-treatment/medications-counseling-related-conditions/naloxone
38. Warner ML, Kaufman NC, Grundmann O. The pharmacology and toxicology of kratom: from traditional herb to drug of abuse. Int J Legal Med. 2016;130(1):127–38.
39. Woo J, Bhalerao A, Bawor M, Bhatt M, Dennis B, Mouravska N, et al. "Don't judge a book its cover": a qualitative study of methadone patients' experiences of stigma. Subst Abuse. 2017;11:1178221816685087.
40. Huhn AS, Dunn KE. Why aren't physicians prescribing more buprenorphine? J Subst Abus Treat. 2017;78:1–7.
41. Providers Clinical Support System. Waiver training for physicians rhode Island. Available from: https://pcssnow.org/medications-for-addiction-treatment/waiver-training-for-physicians/
42. Andrilla CHA, Moore TE, Patterson DG, Larson EH. Geographic distribution of providers with a DEA waiver to prescribe buprenorphine for the treatment of opioid use disorder: a 5-year update. J Rural Health. 2019;35(1):108–12.
43. Velander JR. Suboxone: rationale, science, misconceptions. Ochsner J. 2018;18(1):23–9.

44. Netherland J, Hansen H. White opioids: pharmaceutical race and the war on drugs that wasn't. BioSocieties. 2017;12(2):217–38.
45. Clark RE, Samnaliev M, Baxter JD, Leung GY. The evidence doesn't justify steps by state Medicaid programs to restrict opioid addiction treatment with buprenorphine. Health Aff (Millwood). 2011;30(8):1425–33.
46. Dutra L, Stathopoulou G, Basden SL, Leyro TM, Powers MB, Otto MW. A meta-analytic review of psychosocial interventions for substance use disorders. Am J Psychiatry. 2008;165(2):179–87.
47. Dugosh K, Abraham A, Seymour B, McLoyd K, Chalk M, Festinger D. A systematic review on the use of psychosocial interventions in conjunction with medications for the treatment of opioid addiction. J Addict Med. 2016;10(2):93–103.
48. Carroll KM, Onken LS. Behavioral therapies for drug abuse. Am J Psychiatry. 2005;162(8):1452–60.
49. U.S. Department of Health and Human Services, Substance Abuse and Mental Health Services Administration, Center for Behavioral Health Statistics and Quality. Associations of nonmedical pain reliever use and initiation of heroin use in the United States 2013. Available from: https://www.samhsa.gov/data/sites/default/files/DR006/DR006/nonmedical-pain-reliever-use-2013.htm
50. King JB, Sainski-Nguyen AM, Bellows BK. Office-based buprenorphine versus clinic-based methadone: a cost-effectiveness analysis. J Pain Palliat Care Pharmacother. 2016;30(1):55–65.
51. Schwartz RP, Kelly SM, Mitchell SG, Gryczynski J, O'Grady KE, Jaffe JH. When does methadone treatment reduce arrest and severity of arrest charges? An analysis of arrest records. Drug Alcohol Depend. 2017;180:385–90.
52. Noormohammadi A, Forinash A, Yancey A, Crannage E, Campbell K, Shyken J. Buprenorphine versus methadone for opioid dependence in pregnancy. Ann Pharmacother. 2016;50(8):666–72.
53. Katz DF, Sun J, Khatri V, Kao D, Bucher-Bartelson B, Traut C, et al. QTc interval screening in an opioid treatment program. Am J Cardiol. 2013;112(7):1013–8.
54. Bliesener N, Albrecht S, Schwager A, Weckbecker K, Lichtermann D, Klingmuller D. Plasma testosterone and sexual function in men receiving buprenorphine maintenance for opioid dependence. J Clin Endocrinol Metab. 2005;90(1):203–6.
55. U.S. Department of Health and Human Services, Substance Abuse and Mental Health Services Administration, Buprenorphine; 2020. Available from: https://www.samhsa.gov/medication-assisted-treatment/medications-counseling-related-conditions/buprenorphine

# 8 Sedative-, Hypnotic-, or Anxiolytic-Related Disorders

Emily Dumas

## Introduction

Sedative, hypnotic, and anxiolytic substances include benzodiazepines, barbiturates, and non-benzodiazepine hypnotics. Phenobarbital was introduced in 1912, but due to its potential for toxicity and abuse, was largely supplanted by the benzodiazepines, when chlordiazepoxide came into existence in the early 1960s [5, 13]. The non-benzodiazepines, the so-called Z-drugs, are a newer class, initially thought to occupy a lower level of abuse liability than benzodiazepines, though it has since been demonstrated that they too pose a significant risk of dependence.

The clearest indications for benzodiazepines are in panic disorder, generalized and social anxiety disorders, simple phobias, and for short-term use in acute anxiety and acute insomnia. They are also utilized as the core treatment of alcohol withdrawal in the inpatient setting. It has been estimated that up to 50% of regular benzodiazepine users will experience clinically significant signs of withdrawal with sudden discontinuation [21]. Dose-dependent side effects of benzodiazepines include drowsiness, lethargy, fatigue, sedation, disturbances in concentration and attention, development of dependence, and rebound of insomnia or anxiety after lowering doses [2]. The Z-drugs come with their own set of adverse experiences such as anterograde amnesia, somnambulism, difficulty acquiring new learning, agitation, and hallucinations [4]. Currently, benzodiazepines are considered relatively safe for short-term use in most populations, but their safety has not been established beyond two to four weeks of treatment.

The number of benzodiazepine prescriptions in the United States has increased substantially since the mid-1990s [1, 19]. Dependence develops in approximately half of patients who use benzodiazepines for longer than 1 month [6, 13]. High-risk groups for developing dependence include those with chronic pain syndromes,

E. Dumas (✉)
PGY-2 Psychiatry Resident, Weill Cornell Medical College, New York, NY, USA
e-mail: esd9012@nyp.org



J. D. Avery, D. Hankins (eds.), *Addiction Medicine*, Psychiatry Update 2,
https://doi.org/10.1007/978-3-030-86430-9_8

alcohol or opioid use disorders, chronic sleep disorders, or personality disorders [19]. Additionally, females have an elevated risk of dependence [4]. Among those prescribed benzodiazepines for psychiatric disorders, individuals with anxiety disorders are not as likely to develop use disorders compared to those with affective disorders [4]. Sedative-hypnotic use disorders can also be associated with other substance use disorders, as substance users will often turn to sedatives to mitigate undesirable side effects of other substances or to use synergistically with their primary substance of abuse for mood enhancement. For example, studies have shown that approximately 15–20% of alcoholic patients presenting for treatment may be abusing benzodiazepines [4].

Understanding the mechanism of action of benzodiazepines is critical to grasping their clinical effects, side effects, and pathways to development of a use disorder. The agents in the sedative-hypnotics class have similar mechanisms of action in that they bind to allosteric sites on the gamma-aminobutyric acid subtype A ($GABA_A$) receptor, increasing the frequency of the chloride channel opening. This results in enhancing the inhibitory effect of GABA, translating to the clinical effects of decreased anxiety, increased sedation, muscle relaxation, amnesia, hypnosis, and anticonvulsion [19]. Long-term benzodiazepine use leads to tolerance through downregulation of GABA receptors and upregulation of the excitatory glutamate system [11]. More recent findings show that benzodiazepines may increase the activity of dopaminergic neurons in the ventral tegmental area (VTA), indicating that benzodiazepines may have a mechanism in common with opioids in terms of dopamine release [19]. The benzodiazepines that have the greatest abuse potential have a quick onset of action due to their lipophilicity, enabling them to produce hedonic effects rapidly [6].

Within both the patient and clinician populations, there are barriers to recognizing patterns of misuse and thus diagnosing sedative-hypnotic use disorders. In contrast to opioid intoxication and alcohol withdrawal, benzodiazepines, when ingested alone or being withdrawn from, are rarely fatal. As a result, misuse of these benzodiazepines, in contrast to opioids or alcohol, does not often draw as intensive interventions and treatments. Additionally, sedative, hypnotic, and anxiolytic use disorders are often iatrogenic, arising in the setting of benzodiazepines being taken in doses within the therapeutic range, causing both the prescriber and patient to not view use patterns as problematic. Additionally, some clinicians believe that benzodiazepines are more effective than first-line pharmacologic and nonpharmacologic approaches for insomnia and anxiety, and certain individuals, in particular older people, are less willing to try alternative, more labor-intensive treatments such as cognitive behavioral therapy (CBT). This unwillingness to consider reducing or discontinuing benzodiazepines for an alternative treatment method, along with there being limited resources for alternative treatments such as CBT, leads to benzodiazepine use disorders going unaddressed [8, 15].

The clinical case in this chapter will illustrate many of the key points about benzodiazepine use disorder, highlighting the signs and symptoms of dependence and withdrawal. The case will also give cause for further discussion about how to prescribe and taper benzodiazepines while being mindful of the challenges of achieving abstinence.

## Clinical Case

Dr. Smith is a psychiatry resident in her second year of training, rotating through the Consultation-Liaison Psychiatry service at a hospital in a large urban area. On Dr. Smith's list of consults for the day is a 43-year-old woman, Maya, admitted to a general medicine floor for management of altered mental status. She has a history of generalized anxiety disorder, depression, and anorexia nervosa, in remission, but no significant past medical history. She has been treated by outpatient psychiatrists for a decade. When Maya started seeing her current outpatient psychiatrist two years ago, she was on a regimen consisting of multiple benzodiazepines, including alprazolam, clonazepam, and lorazepam (exact amounts unknown). Since being under the care of her current psychiatrist, Maya's medication regimen has been consolidated to alprazolam 1 mg daily and clonazepam 6.5 mg daily.

Maya was brought by ambulance to the hospital's emergency after her outpatient psychiatrist noticed that earlier that day, during their weekly virtual check-in appointment, Maya presented as disorganized, inattentive, and not oriented to time or place. Upon this evaluation, Maya slurred her speech, exhibited paranoid delusions (e.g., she accused her psychiatrist of posting about her on social media), and reported having not slept in three days. Per collateral from Maya's parents, who live in Florida, Maya started behaving bizarrely four days ago, when she sent several aggressively worded text messages to her father, which was uncharacteristic of her.

After Maya was admitted to the medicine floor, the primary team of doctors initiated an altered mental status workup, including a metabolic panel, ammonia level, carboxyhemoglobin level, and head imaging, none of which had pathological findings. Additionally, Maya's urine toxicology screen and blood alcohol level were insignificant. The primary team gave her fluids and placed orders for a Clinical Institute Withdrawal Assessment (CIWA) to be completed every four hours to monitor for benzodiazepine withdrawal.

When Dr. Smith first came to see Maya the day following her admission, Maya presented as a thin woman lying calmly in bed who appeared stated age, but was disheveled and displayed limited eye contact. Maya reported a "scared" mood and had an anxious affect. Her thought process was linear but vague. No paranoia, delusions, or perceptual disturbances were elicited in her thought content. She denied auditory and visual hallucinations. Maya explained that she had not taken her alprazolam or clonazepam in over a week because she had abruptly run out of pills and could not manage to get them refilled for unclear reasons. Maya did not recall sending text messages to her father or speaking with her psychiatrist the day she was brought to the emergency department.

Dr. Smith recommended starting Maya on clonazepam 1.5 mg every 8 h in the hospital, to be held for sedation, and keeping Maya on CIWA for benzodiazepine withdrawal precautions. After two days in the hospital, Maya became clearer and cognitively intact. She denied using any illicit substances, though admitted that in the last few months she was drinking alone more often, consuming at least one or two glasses of wine most nights, and sometimes up to a bottle of wine on a weekend. She explained that the social isolation she was experiencing was making her anxious, so she took it upon herself to self-medicate with tablets of alprazolam and clonazepam every day. She recalled that approximately one day after she ran out of her benzodiazepine prescriptions, she began to experience heightened anxiety, irritability, and confusion. She described feeling as though she were in a fog and having an "out of body experience." During this time, she stopped running her usual daily six miles. Maya discussed multiple life stressors including her father's recent diagnosis with lymphoma, her dog's illness, migraines, and social isolation in the setting of the pandemic, compounded by the loss of her job in the setting of layoffs early in the pandemic. Her mother, who had arrived in the city by time of discharge, was planning on staying with her for at least the next couple of weeks. The discharge plan was for Maya to follow up with her outpatient psychiatrist the next day.

## Discussion

Maya's initial presentation was consistent with delirium secondary to benzodiazepine withdrawal, in the setting of benzodiazepine use disorder. Within days of suddenly stopping her benzodiazepines, Maya experienced a concurrent acute change in mental status, marked by escalating confusion, disorientation, and memory impairment. This evolved into disorganization and frank psychosis, as evidenced by her paranoia that her psychiatrist was posting about her on social media. The differential diagnosis included benzodiazepine or alcohol acute intoxication, alcohol withdrawal, and unspecified psychosis.

Maya's delirious presentation was characteristic of the moderate-to-severe withdrawal that is usually experienced by individuals who abruptly stop taking medium-to-high doses of benzodiazepines after regularly taking them for at least two to six months. Maya's outpatient regimen of alprazolam 1 mg and clonazepam 6.5 mg daily, doses approximately equivalent to lorazepam 15 mg daily, was a high amount of benzodiazepines, relative to the average prescriptions of benzodiazepines. The severity and duration of withdrawal is multifactorial, depending upon the potency and half-life of the benzodiazepine, the amount taken, and the duration of use prior to discontinuation. Some sources suggest it may take as little as four weeks of regular use to develop withdrawal symptoms; others report that rebound insomnia can be seen after two weeks of daily use [7, 9]. With shorter half-life agents like alprazolam, symptoms can develop as early as 24 hours after discontinuation, and the severity of withdrawal peaks on average between one and three days. In contrast, for longer half-life agents like clonazepam, symptoms of withdrawal can begin later and peak as late as four to seven days after drug discontinuation [5]. For Maya, who was taking a combination of alprazolam and clonazepam, the onset of withdrawal symptoms is more difficult to predict, but based on her presentation, her withdrawal symptoms likely occurred within one or two days after sudden discontinuation. The withdrawal from short-acting benzodiazepines tends to be experienced as more intense than that associated with long-acting benzodiazepines, but indeed, there is variability in the sensitivity of individuals to discontinuation. Variation among individuals is dependent upon several factors, including any that influence the metabolism of drugs, such as age and medical health. Furthermore, underlying psychopathology, for example, Maya's depression and anxiety, can elevate the severity of the withdrawal symptoms. Conversely, when benzodiazepines are administered for short periods and at therapeutic doses, the withdrawal syndrome is usually mild, consisting of anxiety, headache, insomnia, dysphoria, and tremor or muscle twitching. In individuals experiencing acute withdrawal like Maya, pharmacologic management is often recommended because of the risk of serious consequences, including seizures and delirium tremens. Thus, Maya was placed on standing benzodiazepines (clonazepam 1.5 mg every eight hours) as well as CIWA precautions, which would have also protected her had she been experiencing alcohol withdrawal, a syndrome that can mimic the appearance of benzodiazepine withdrawal. It is worth noting that the abrupt discontinuation of barbiturates, in contrast to that of benzodiazepines or alcohol, has the greatest propensity to result in severe symptoms, including grand mal seizures [7]. As such, barbiturates are considered less safe and tolerable than benzodiazepines, and thus the prescription of benzodiazepines has largely replaced that of barbiturates for inducing sleep and anxiolysis.

Maya's history of depression, anxiety, and an eating disorder made her vulnerable to developing benzodiazepine dependence. The risk of dependence on benzodiazepines is associated with a history of mental illness and with higher doses of drugs taken [10]. The greatest risk factors for benzodiazepine dependence include a longer duration of treatment with these agents, treatment at higher doses, and concurrent substance misuse [3, 12].

Among individuals who abuse substances, it is uncommon for benzodiazepines to be the primary drug of use [7]. Individuals with current or remote alcohol and/or opioid use disorders comprise two groups with high rates of benzodiazepine abuse-related problems. Concurrent use of other substances, such as opioids or stimulants, can conflate or exacerbate the benzodiazepine withdrawal and intoxication presentation, as their intoxication syndromes can present similarly with impaired motor performance and sedation. If a clinician suspects opioid use in a patient who has altered mental status, naloxone can be administered without any negative repercussions. Although Maya's blood alcohol level was negligible on her admission labs, her increased alcohol intake in recent months should be addressed in subsequent treatment to prevent a potentially fatal overdose if she were to combine alcohol with benzodiazepines. Such poor outcomes underscore the importance that clinicians screen for benzodiazepine use in patients with co-occurring substance use disorders [7].

Lower on the differential for Maya's clinical presentation was intoxication with benzodiazepines or alcohol, as well as other metabolic disturbances, given that her metabolic panel, blood alcohol level, and urine toxicology screen were unremarkable. Severe toxicity with benzodiazepines can manifest, in the most severe cases, as stupor, coma, respiratory arrest, or cardiovascular collapse [7]. Management in severely intoxicated patients is largely supportive, with the goal of maintaining the airway. Flumazenil is indicated only in those with confirmed benzodiazepine toxicity who are losing consciousness; however, it has limited use due to its risk of precipitating seizures [5]. Mild-to-moderate acute toxicity of benzodiazepines—which can occur even within a therapeutic context of benzodiazepine use—is characterized by sedation, slurred speech, psychomotor impairment, ataxia, altered visuospatial skills, and memory problems [4]. Maya exhibited lapses in memory, but this was more likely secondary to her delirious state, not necessarily a result of benzodiazepine use. The cognitive side effects of benzodiazepines, such as difficulty with attention, concentration, and acquiring new learning, tend to be insidious, rather than acute [20]. Benzodiazepines, as well as Z-drugs, have the potential to produce acute anterograde amnesia; in fact, impairment of learning new information is a drawback of this class of medications. There is a multitude of documented cases of zolpidem and zaleplon, especially at high doses, being associated with bizarre behaviors like somnambulism and nocturnal eating, shopping, and driving. Tolerance can develop to some of these cognitive effects, but not in all patients, and not always to the same degree. Although benzodiazepines can contribute to cognitive impairment, the association between benzodiazepine use and late-life cognitive disorders such as dementia remains controversial [17].

## Treatment

Benzodiazepine discontinuation plans are heterogeneous; the approach taken is largely determined by the severity of benzodiazepine dependence. Benzodiazepine discontinuation can be managed in either the inpatient setting, where rapid dose reduction may occur, or in the outpatient setting, with close monitoring and a slower taper over weeks to months. Individuals with medical comorbidities, comorbid use of other substances, high-dose sedative-hypnotic use, or extensive mental health issues are best managed in inpatient facilities for detoxification [19]. The outpatient setting is best suited for those with long-term use and physical dependence at therapeutic doses, as well as for individuals who do not have significant comorbid substance use disorders and can reliably present for outpatient appointments.

Prior to determining the discontinuation protocol in an individual, a thorough sedative-hypnotic history is recommended, encompassing the doses taken, the duration of use, and the overall clinical response to these agents throughout the course of use [7]. To complete this history, it is necessary to find out all of the sources from which the individual is obtaining benzodiazepines from, as some individuals may be using a combination of prescribed and non-prescribed benzodiazepines, the latter of which may be related to a form of diversion, such as taken from family members or friends or purchased off the street. It is key for the provider to be cognizant that the prescription monitoring database is not necessarily comprehensive and probe about other avenues of obtaining benzodiazepines. It is also imperative to know which other psychoactive substances are currently being taken, as other substances can conflate the withdrawal picture. This can be further ascertained with regular drug screens at appointments. Prior to discontinuing, it is important to provide psychoeducation, including the reasons for discontinuation, the signs and symptoms likely to be experienced, and the pros and cons of the various withdrawal strategies.

The method of withdrawal considered to be most effective and safe features a fixed taper, usually occurring over a period ranging from 4 to 12 weeks [22]. The taper is extended weeks to months in order to prevent severe withdrawal symptoms such as seizures and delirium. If an individual is using multiple benzodiazepines, as was the case for Maya, the clinician can consolidate to a single agent. More specifically, the clinician may substitute short-acting benzodiazepines (e.g., alprazolam or lorazepam) for longer-acting benzodiazepines (e.g., chlordiazepoxide or clonazepam) at equivalent doses, since longer-acting benzodiazepines minimize the interdose withdrawal symptoms [19]. The dose can then be decreased on a weekly or every-other-week basis over the course of 4–12 weeks [5, 7]. Recommendations range from reducing the initial benzodiazepine dose by 50% approximately every week to reducing by between 10% and 25% every two weeks [19]. Prolonged reductions over many months should be avoided to prevent the withdrawal treatment from becoming the individual's "morbid focus" [14]. Lastly, the rate of withdrawal is often determined by the individuals' ability to tolerate symptoms, but generally, the first 50% of the taper is experienced as smoother and mildly symptomatic, in contrast to the last 50% of the taper [16, 18, 19]. If intolerable symptoms of withdrawal do occur, the dose can be increased slightly until the symptoms resolve. Following the development of intolerable withdrawal symptoms, subsequent dose reductions should be more conservative in terms of amount and speed of reduction [5].

Clinicians conducting benzodiazepine discontinuation should be prepared to manage the emergence of psychiatric disorders—such as insomnia or anxiety—during the withdrawal period. Concomitant psychopharmacotherapy for withdrawal lacks robust evidence, but is generally symptom-based. Medications to mitigate withdrawal symptoms include sleep-inducing agents such as mirtazapine and trazodone, as well as anxiolytic agents such as pregabalin, gabapentin, hydroxyzine, or diphenhydramine [19]. Individuals can also experience a state known as "pseudo-withdrawal," defined as "overinterpretation of symptoms secondary to the expectations of withdrawal" [11]. Additionally, individuals undergoing tapering may experience rebound symptoms, in which their pre-benzodiazepine symptoms of anxiety or insomnia return but are experienced more intensely than their original symptoms were [5]. It is key that clinicians counsel individuals about the variety of potential adverse responses during the withdrawal period and provide reassurance that rebound symptoms usually dissipate or return to original levels within weeks. Additionally, employing psychotherapeutic treatments, such as cognitive behavioral therapy, helps the individual manage psychosocial stress factors and likewise addresses situations that are high risk for relapse [19].

Although benzodiazepines are rarely the first-line treatment for anxiety and sleep disorders, when the first-line approaches fail to control symptoms, benzodiazepines should not be withheld. After trialing first-line treatment modalities, such as cognitive behavioral therapy, group therapy, relaxation therapy, stress management, antidepressants, and buspirone, benzodiazepines may be considered as adjunctive treatments for individuals experiencing refractory anxiety, panic, or phobias, at least for the short term. Particularly important for the aging and elderly in these cases, the goal when administering benzodiazepines is to use the lowest possible dose for the shortest period of time [7]. However, for individuals with current or history of substance use disorder, benzodiazepines should be avoided at all costs due to the higher risk of fatal overdose. If there is uncertainty about how effective a benzodiazepine is for the refractory symptoms once the individual begins taking it, a brief taper can be tried to determine whether continued administration of the benzodiazepine is indeed indicated [16]. When selecting a benzodiazepine agent, one can consider both the potency and pharmacokinetics (e.g., speed of onset and duration of action of the agent). Clinicians should aim to prescribe the lowest potency and longest-acting agents (e.g., clonazepam instead of alprazolam) at the lowest effective doses, because these qualities decrease the abuse potential. See Table 8.1 for a list of commonly used benzodiazepines, their half-lives, and dose equivalencies. In the outpatient setting, clinicians typically prescribe to achieve a steady state, so the critical variable to consider when selecting a benzodiazepine is elimination half-life. In contrast, in the emergency setting, the critical variable is the distribution half-life, with the goal being fastest onset of action.

In order to prevent iatrogenic benzodiazepine dependence when prescribing benzodiazepines, clinicians can check the state's prescription drug monitoring program, available in the vast majority of states in the United States, as this helps to avoid situations in which multiple providers are prescribing controlled substances. Further, clinicians can educate individuals about the regulation of benzodiazepines, specifically about the policies of no early refills and no prescriptions for benzodiazepines from multiple physicians. See Table 8.2 for a list of signs and symptoms of benzodiazepine use disorder. Furthermore, providers should explain that benzodiazepines are viewed as short-term therapies, the need for which will be re-evaluated at frequent intervals and be discontinued as soon as clinical symptoms improve or if the indication changes [7]. In situations that allow for it, family members can be educated about the risks of combining benzodiazepines with opioids or alcohol, since family members are often the first to recognize misuse.

**Table 8.1** Benzodiazepine doses and equivalencies

| Benzodiazepine | Onset after oral dose | Distribution half-life | Elimination half-life (h) | Dose equivalency |
|---|---|---|---|---|
| Diazepam (Valium) | Fastest | Fast | Slow (30–100 h) | 5 mg |
| Lorazepam (Ativan) | Fast (IV), intermediate (PO) | Intermediate | Fast (10–20 h) | 1 mg |
| Alprazolam (Xanax) | Intermediate-fast | Intermediate | Fast (6–20 h) | 0.5 mg |
| Clonazepam (Klonopin) | Intermediate | Intermediate | Intermediate (18–50 h) | 0.25 mg |

**Table 8.2** Signs and symptoms of sedative-, hypnotic-, and anxiolytic-related use disorders

| |
|---|
| History of sedative overdose |
| History of or current prescription misuse |
| History of taking benzodiazepines for years, especially with history of increasing dose instead of tapering |
| History of "doctor shopping" as evidenced by multiple providers listed in prescription monitoring database |
| History of emergency room visits for prescriptions |
| Concurrent substance misuse |
| Patient initially reporting improvement in anxiety symptoms and at a later date seeking to increase dose for anxiety |
| Patient reporting lost or stolen prescriptions >1 time |
| Patient refusal to accept alternative non-benzodiazepine treatments (e.g., buspirone, pregabalin, antidepressant, hydroxyzine, CBT) for anxiety |

## Conclusion

Sedative-, hypnotic, and anxiolytic-related disorders can develop in a variety of individuals, including those taking them at therapeutic doses for anxiety or phobia disorders, as well as those seeking them for different motives, such as mood enhancement or to mitigate unwanted side effects from other substance misuse. The withdrawal symptoms are often experienced as unpleasant if not intolerable, and a monitored discontinuation protocol is the optimal management for long-term success in overcoming a use disorder. Individuals taking these agents must be educated about the signs of dependence and symptoms of withdrawal prior to initiating their use. If the medications are prescribed at reasonable doses for limited periods of time, sedative hypnotics can be used safely and effectively to treat severe anxiety, panic, and phobia disorders.

### Key Points

- For individuals prescribed with benzodiazepines, the continued need for these medications should be reassessed on a regular basis.
- Benzodiazepine withdrawal can be inadvertently initiated by a physician due to concerns of misuse, dependence, or co-occurring substance use disorders.
- For discontinuation of benzodiazepines, the consensus is a slow taper over a period of 4–12 weeks, largely dependent upon the individual's ability to tolerate dose reduction.
- Clinicians should discuss the risks in prescribing sedative hypnotics, such as dependence and withdrawal, and counsel individuals about benzodiazepines' potentially lethal interactions with other substances such as opioids and alcohol.

## References


1. Bachhuber MA, Henessy S, Cunningham CO, Starrels JL. Increasing benzodiazepine prescriptions and overdose mortality in the United States, 1996–2013. Am J Public Health. 2016;106:686–8.
2. Buffett-Jerrott SE, Stewart SH. Cognitive and sedative effects of benzodiazepine use. Curr Pharm Des. 2002;8:45–58.
3. Busto UE, Romach MK, Sellers EM. Multiple drug use and psychiatric comorbidity in patients admitted to the hospital with severe benzodiazepine dependence. J Clin Psychopharmacol. 1996;16(1):51–7.
4. Ciraulo DA, Knapp CM. The pharmacology of nonalcohol sedative hypnotics. In: Ries RK, Fiellin DA, Miller SC, Saitz R, editors. The ASAM principles of addiction medicine. Philadelphia: Lippincott Williams & Wilkins; 2014.
5. Cluver JS, Wright TM, Myick H. Pharmacologic intervention for sedative-hypnotic addiction. In: Ries RK, Fiellin DA, Miller SC, Saitz R, editors. The ASAM principles of addiction medicine. Philadelphia: Lippincott Williams & Wilkins; 2014. p. 727–33.
6. De las Cuevas C, Sanz E, de la Fuente J. Benzodiazepines: more "behavioral" addiction than dependence. Psychopharmacology. 2003;167:297–303.
7. Dickinson WE, Eickelberg SJ. Management of sedative-hypnotic intoxication and withdrawal. In: Ries RK, Fiellin DA, Miller SC, Saitz R, editors. The ASAM principles of addiction medicine. Philadelphia: Lippincott Williams & Wilkins; 2014.
8. Everitt H, McDermott L, Leydon G, Yules H, Baldwin D, Little P. GPs' management strategies for patients with insomnia: a survey and qualitative interview study. Br J Gen Pract. 2014;64(619):e112–0.
9. Fontaine R, Chouinard G, Annable L. Rebound anxiety in anxious patients after abrupt withdrawal of benzodiazepine treatment. Am J Psychiatry. 1984;141:848–52.
10. Guerlais M, Grall-Bronnec M, Feuillet F, Gerardin M, Joliet P, Victorri-Vigneau C. Dependence on prescription benzodiazepines and Z-drugs among young to middle-aged patients in France. Subst Use Misuse. 2015;50:320–7.
11. Kalira V. Benzodiazepines. In: Levounis P, Zerbo E, Aggarwal R, editors. Pocket guide to addiction assessment and treatment. 1st ed. Arlington: American Psychiatric Assoc Publishing; 2016. p. 81–96.
12. Kan CC, Hilberink SR, Breteler MH. Determination of the main risk factors for benzodiazepine dependence using a multivariate and multidimensional approach. Compr Psychiatry. 2004;45(2):88–94.
13. Lader M. Benzodiazepines revisited – will we ever learn? Addiction. 2011;106:2086–109.
14. Lader M, Tylee A, Donogue J. Withdrawing benzodiazepines in primary care. CNS Drugs. 2009;23:19–34.
15. Olfston M, King M, Schoenbaum M. Benzodiazepine use in the United States. JAMA Psychiat. 2015;72:136–42.
16. Rickels K, DeMartinis N, Rynn M. Pharmacologic strategies for discontinuing benzodiazepine treatment. J Clin Psychopharmacol. 1999;19(6 Suppl 2):12S–6S.
17. Salzman C. Do benzodiazepines cause Alzheimer's disease? Am J Psychiatry. 2020;177(6):476–8. https://doi.org/10.1176/appi.ajp.2020.20040375.
18. Schweizer E, Rickels K, Case G. Long-term therapeutic use of benzodiazepines: effects of gradual taper. Arch Gen Psychiatry. 1990;47:908.
19. Soyka M. Treatment of benzodiazepine dependence. N Engl J Med. 2017;376:1147–57.
20. Stewart SA. The effects of benzodiazepines on cognition. J Clin Psychiatry. 2005;66(Suppl 2):9–13.
21. Tyrer P. Benzodiazepine dependence: a shadowy diagnosis. Biochem Soc Symp. 1993;59:107–19.
22. Voshaar RC, Couvee JE, van Balkom AJ. Strategies for discontinuing long-term benzodiazepine use: meta-analysis. Br J Psychiatry. 2006;189:213–20.

# Stimulant-Related Disorders

# 9

Matthew Boyer

## Introduction

The substances of abuse in stimulant-related disorders include cocaine, methamphetamine, amphetamines, and synthetic cathinones. Users enjoy stimulants because of the effects of euphoria, increased energy, and elevated libido stimulants can bring about. The stimulant withdrawal syndrome, known as a crash, can be marked by dysphoria and hypersomnia. For many users, withdrawal can be unpleasant enough to trigger cravings for continued use of stimulants. Cravings, in turn, can lead to repeated use of stimulants, paving the way to development of a stimulant-related disorder.

Data from a national survey in the United States show that about 977,000 people aged 12 or older met criteria in 2018 for cocaine use disorder [1]. More people use cocaine than any other illegal drug in the United States aside from cannabis, with an additional four million people using cocaine in the past year but not meeting criteria for a use disorder [2]. Prevalence of cocaine use is highest among white men in their 20s, those who were previously married, those unemployed, those living in nonrural areas, and those who did not complete high school [3].

About 1.1 million people aged 12 or older met criteria in 2018 for methamphetamine use disorder [1]. It has been reported that 4.7 million Americans have tried methamphetamine at some point in their lives [4]. Men have been found to have a higher three-year prevalence rate than women [5]. In the United States, rates of methamphetamine use have historically been highest in the western and mid-western regions [6].

About 561,000 people aged 12 or older met criteria in 2018 for prescription stimulant use disorder [1]. Amphetamines are prescribed for several conditions, including attention-deficit/hyperactivity disorder, narcolepsy, and weight loss. Diversion of prescribed amphetamines can contribute to misuse and abuse of

M. Boyer (✉)
Psychiatrist, Rogers Behavioral Health, Philadelphia, PA, USA
e-mail: matthew.boyer@rogersbh.org



J. D. Avery, D. Hankins (eds.), *Addiction Medicine*, Psychiatry Update 2,
https://doi.org/10.1007/978-3-030-86430-9_9

amphetamines. An estimated 5.3 million people in the United States had misused prescription stimulants within the preceding year [2]. Measures have been taken to create long-acting formulations of prescribed stimulants to lower their potential for abuse.

Use of synthetic cathinones (bath salts) is much lower in prevalence compared to that of the other three types of stimulants.

Patients with stimulant-related disorders can present for care in the outpatient setting or be admitted to an inpatient unit for treatment. For example, patients can present to ambulatory substance abuse clinics on their own volition, with encouragement from loved ones, or be referred there by the courts. Patients with stimulant-related disorders can also present to emergency departments and then be admitted to inpatient units. For example, during the intoxication phase, some stimulant users can become aggressive or experience psychosis characterized by paranoid ideation and auditory hallucinations. During the withdrawal phase, dysphoria can be so profound that some stimulant users present to emergency departments with suicidal ideation. In the case described next, emergency medical services were activated for a patient expressing homicidal ideation while intoxicated on methamphetamine.

## Clinical Case

Simon is a 30-year-old man who has sex with men and has no prior psychiatric history. Emergency medical services transported Simon from his home to the emergency department after his roommate called 911 to report that Simon was making homicidal comments.

Upon entering the patient's room in the emergency department, Simon is observed to be talking to himself. On interview, the patient describes a scheme whereby his neighbor has hacked his webcam to intercept private masturbation videos he shares on a group sex website. Simon says there is evidence to support the notion that he's been hacked. For example, he notices delays when he livestreams his videos. Sometimes, he says, the videos fail to stream altogether. He reports that his neighbor is using a "data beam" she has aimed through his window into his apartment in order to intercept his videos. The patient reports hearing his neighbor speaking to him at the time of the interview.

Collateral is obtained from the roommate who called 911. The roommate says that the patient has been fixated on a window in the patient's room at home. The roommate recalls that Simon first put up tin foil to cover the window for no apparent reason. He then moved a heavy bookshelf in front of the window to block the window altogether. Asked what happened that the roommate decided to call 911, the roommate says the patient started repeating "I'm going to kill her" and was pacing anxiously in their small apartment. The roommate states that the patient in recent weeks has been smoking increasing amounts of "tina," not sleeping, and hardly eating.

On mental status exam, the patient is malnourished, and his hair is unkempt. Thought content is notable for delusions of persecution. Perceptual disturbances are present, notably auditory hallucinations. The patient's speech is rapid but interruptible, and his thought process is linear. He is alert and grossly oriented. On workup, labs and electrocardiogram (EKG) are unremarkable. Simon's urine toxicology is positive for methamphetamine when the results came back a short time later.

The treating physician suspects a stimulant-related disorder based on the presenting history and objective findings. Given the severity of Simon's psychosis, Simon is admitted to the inpatient psychiatric service. Provided below is additional discussion about Simon's case and treatment.

## Discussion

Simon is having auditory hallucinations and delusions of persecution in the setting of increased use of methamphetamine. His psychosis is most likely substance-induced. Also on the differential is a psychotic disorder such as schizophrenia. Psychosis in the setting of stimulant abuse can present a diagnostic challenge; stimulant-induced psychosis is sometimes misdiagnosed as schizophrenia [7]. Diagnostic ambiguity can be compounded by the fact that some individuals with chronic psychotic disorders also have stimulant use disorders. In this case, however, schizophrenia is less likely than methamphetamine-induced psychosis because of the relatively acute onset of symptoms in a patient with no known prior history of psychotic symptoms. Additional features of the case making schizophrenia less likely are the patient's linear thought process and the absence of negative symptoms.

Episodes of methamphetamine-induced psychosis typically are short-lived, although for some, episodes have been known to last six months or longer [8]. Even though they were not present in Simon's presentation, tactile hallucinations are common in stimulant-induced psychosis, especially formication (the sensation that insects are crawling under or on one's skin). When patients present in the intoxication phase, stimulant users typically have intact orientation.

Workup should include urine toxicology to evaluate for other potential substances of abuse. Labs should be ordered to rule out possible medical explanations for the patient's presentation, such as hyperthyroidism or hypoglycemia. Workup should also include EKG due to risk for cardiac arrhythmias. Physical exam should include evaluation of injection sites for signs of infection if patients are using intravenously.

Aside from methamphetamine-induced psychosis, the patient also meets criteria for methamphetamine use disorder based on additional history gathered from the patient during his hospitalization. For example, Simon later reported problematic use of methamphetamine for the previous two years. His problematic use had been marked by an inability to cut back on his use of methamphetamine, having cravings to use methamphetamine, losing two jobs in the catering industry due to his methamphetamine use, and experiencing both tolerance and withdrawal. He also admitted that his use in recent months had escalated from smoking methamphetamine to injecting it and to using more than he had intended.

**Table 9.1** Stimulants and their street names, routes of administration, and effects of intoxication and withdrawal

| Substance | Street names | Routes of administration | Intoxication | Withdrawal |
|---|---|---|---|---|
| Cocaine | Coke, snow, blow | Intranasal, smoking, injection, suppository | Euphoria, increased energy, heightened alertness, increased sociability, decreased need for sleep, poor appetite. The intoxication phase can also include unwanted effects such as anxiety, irritability, hypervigilance, suspiciousness, grandiosity, stereotyped behaviors, delusions, and hallucinations | Dysphoria, anhedonia, fatigue, poor concentration, hypersomnolence, increased dreaming, increased appetite, arthralgias, chills, tremors, and involuntary motor movements |
| Methamphetamine | Crystal, tina, ice, speed | Oral, intranasal, smoking, injection | | |
| Amphetamine | Addys, smart pills | Oral, intranasal | | |
| Synthetic cathinones | Bath salts, cloud nine, vanilla sky | Oral, intranasal, smoking, injecting | | |

The substance of methamphetamine itself can take on the physical appearance of shards of glass. Hence, it is commonly referred to as crystal meth. It is also known on the street as “speed,” “ice,” “crank,” “glass,” or “tina.” Methamphetamine and other stimulants have sympathomimetic effects. The increase in catecholamine neurotransmitter activity has downstream physical effects, including tachycardia, tachypnea, hyperthermia, hypertension, and anorexia. Psychiatrically, patients can experience anxiety, insomnia, or, as seen in Simon’s case, psychosis. Withdrawal from stimulants can include dysphoria, increased appetite, and hypersomnia. See Table 9.1.

In light of the struggles he has been experiencing personally and professionally now culminating in a hospitalization for psychosis, Simon could benefit from a number of available pharmacologic and nonpharmacologic treatment options.

## Treatment

While on the inpatient unit, Simon was started on risperidone, and the dose was titrated to 2 mg at nighttime. Simon’s symptoms of psychosis resolved quickly. Because of some evidence demonstrating that mirtazapine can be helpful in patients with methamphetamine use disorder, the patient was started on mirtazapine on an off-label basis and titrated to a nighttime dose of 30 mg. The patient reported tolerating both risperidone and mirtazapine well. Inpatient treatment lasted for six days. The patient’s social worker lined up an intake appointment for the patient at the treating hospital’s affiliated chemical dependency outpatient clinic. Unfortunately, he did not present for that appointment. When contacted by telephone for post-hospitalization tracking, the patient stated he was no longer taking either the risperidone or the mirtazapine. He said he had returned to using methamphetamine, albeit reportedly in doses smaller than he had previously been using. He declined re-referral to outpatient substance treatment.

When treating patients with stimulant-related disorders, it is important to identify goals of treatment. Reduction or elimination of psychotic symptoms, return to school or re-entry into the workforce, maintaining abstinence from any stimulant use, and merely cutting back on stimulant use are goals worth discussing with patients.

In Simon's case, had he followed up with outpatient care, the treating psychiatrist would have needed to talk to him about the use of the antipsychotic. Long-term treatment with an antipsychotic is not required in cases of methamphetamine-induced psychosis if the symptoms of psychosis remit. An antipsychotic should only be prescribed to a patient with methamphetamine-induced psychosis who is still experiencing psychosis or who has had less than 3–6 months of stability on the antipsychotic. If the patient is psychiatrically stable after six months of use of an antipsychotic, the psychiatrist should consider tapering off the antipsychotic with continued close monitoring of the patient. Long-term treatment with an antipsychotic in resolved methamphetamine-induced psychosis is not indicated.

Unlike tobacco, opioid, and alcohol use disorders for which treatment options include FDA-approved medications, there is no FDA-approved medication for treatment of stimulant-related disorders. Simon was started on mirtazapine on an off-label basis. The rationale for prescribing mirtazapine was based on a study showing that men who have sex with men (MSM) prescribed mirtazapine had decreased use of methamphetamine [9]. The number needed to treat was 3.1. An expanded replication trial showed that the addition of mirtazapine in methamphetamine users reduced methamphetamine use as well as some human immunodeficiency virus (HIV) risk [10]. Another study has shown that more patients with methamphetamine use disorder responded to the combination of extended-release injectable naltrexone plus oral extended-release bupropion than those given placebo [11]. The number needed to treat was nine. Regarding cocaine use disorder research, the combination of extended release mixed amphetamine salts and topiramate has been found to be efficacious in promoting abstinence among adults with cocaine use disorder [12].

In the absence of an FDA-approved medication for stimulant-related disorders, psychotherapeutic approaches are critical. Several psychotherapeutic modalities have demonstrated efficacy. Drug counseling consists of individual and group sessions that center around topics of education and recovery. Drug counseling has demonstrated efficacy in reducing cocaine use among people with cocaine use disorder [13]. Cognitive behavioral therapy (CBT) has been shown to be efficacious in patients with cocaine use disorder [14] and methamphetamine use disorder [15]. CBT can be used to build skills helpful in maintaining abstinence [16]. See Table 9.2 for a sample of coping skills useful in the management of cravings for substances. Because of the link between stimulant-related disorders and high-risk sexual

**Table 9.2** A sample of coping skills useful in the management of cravings for substances

| Skill | Comment |
|---|---|
| Urge surfing [22] | Cravings peak and then pass. Patients practice imagining themselves surfing on a large wave |
| Distraction [23] | Patients identify activities (especially physical activities) to engage in to distract them from intense urges to use |
| Recall of negative consequences [23] | Patients practice asking themselves, "How do I feel the day after using?" "What effect does using have on my relationships?" |
| Talking about craving [23] | Sharing the burden of cravings with a confidant or sponsor can offer relief. Patients can call an anonymous helpline (1-800-622-HELP) if a supportive contact is not available |
| Using self-talk [23] | Using positive rather than negative self-talk to challenge automatic thoughts about cravings and the perceived urgency to use |
| Normalize [23] | Patients practice recognizing that cravings are uncomfortable, expected, and can be experienced without resorting to use |

**Table 9.3** Motivational interviewing [24] concepts and examples of questions

| Concept | Examples of possible questions |
|---|---|
| Open-ended questions | "Tell me about your use of crystal meth."<br>"What are the benefits of using cocaine?" |
| Affirmations | "I see how hard you're working at cutting back."<br>"You're demonstrating good insight about your triggers to use." |
| Reflections | "You sense there may be a connection between your moods and your use of cocaine."<br>"You've noticed more conflict with your partner when you exceed the prescribed dose of your stimulant medication." |
| Summary statements | "Let me make sure I understand. You just explained how…." |

behavior in MSM, some treatment programs include a concurrent focus on addressing high-risk sexual behaviors.

Other interventions include contingency management and aerobic exercise. Contingency management has demonstrated efficacy among patients with stimulant-related disorders in maintaining abstinence from stimulants [17]. Contingency management is a behavioral intervention used to augment other psychotherapeutic interventions. It relies on rewards to incentivize attainment of treatment goals. Voucher reinforcement and intermittent prize reinforcement are two strategies used in contingency management. Data also support implementing a program of aerobic exercise in patients with methamphetamine use disorder [18].

Employment of the tenets of motivational interviewing when speaking to patients with stimulant-related disorders is helpful. Maintenance of a non-judgmental stance with patients who abuse stimulants can build an alliance and foster openness. A strong alliance and openness may be features of treatment especially important to patients who experience shame or face stigma. When gathering a history, it can be helpful to normalize behaviors. For example, you might try asking the following, "Some people enjoy crystal meth because it is known to enhance sexual experiences.

I am curious to understand the ways crystal meth affects your sex life." Also ask about other substances with which stimulant users may be inclined to experiment or abuse, including gamma-hydroxybutyrate (GHB), 3,4-methylenedioxymethamphetamine (MDMA), and ketamine. Use the principles of motivational interviewing. See Table 9.3 for motivational interviewing concepts and examples.

Harm reduction is an important strategy to employ in patients with stimulant-related disorders for at least two reasons. First, relapse is common. In the case of methamphetamine use disorder, the relapse rate is 61% within the first 12 months [19]. The second reason that harm reduction is important in stimulant-related disorders is that stimulants in high doses can be cardiotoxic. Harm reduction can help to mitigate risks from relapse. In keeping with a harm-reduction approach, try to ask patients presenting with stimulant-related disorders about sex work, condomless sex, routine screening for sexually transmitted illnesses (STIs), and pre-exposure prophylaxis (PrEP) to decrease the risk for HIV. Patients should be referred for STI screening along with screening for PrEP (or post-exposure prophylaxis, if indicated). Speedballing, the practice of combining a stimulant with an opioid, puts patients with stimulant-related disorders at risk for opioid overdoses. For this reason, it is appropriate to educate patients with stimulant-related disorders about the use of naloxone and to prescribe naloxone as a harm-reduction measure.

Some patients diagnosed with stimulant-related disorders suffer from comorbid psychiatric illness. For example, among patients with methamphetamine use disorder, 16% have a comorbid mood disorder and 7% have a comorbid anxiety disorder [20]. A tenet of treatment of stimulant-related disorders – and of substance use disorders more broadly – is to optimize treatment of any comorbid psychiatric disorders. Providers should also be careful to consider the role of early-life trauma. Early-life trauma has been shown to affect treatment success in methamphetamine use disorder [21].

Finally, support services are available. The Substance Abuse and Mental Health Services Administration (SAMHSA) operates a national helpline for people interested in referrals for substance treatment. The number is 1-800-662-HELP. Crystal Meth Anonymous is a 12-step recovery program. It runs a 24-hour helpline at 1-855-Meth-Free (1-855-638-4373). The organization's website (https://www.crystalmeth.org/) has a map feature to help patients find local meetings. Cocaine Anonymous is another option for patients with stimulant-related disorders.

## Conclusion

The substances of abuse in stimulant-related disorders include cocaine, methamphetamine, amphetamines, and synthetic cathinones. Mental health workers aware of patients abusing stimulants should assess whether patients meet criteria for a stimulant-related disorder and screen for abuse of other substances. Although there is no FDA-approved medication for stimulant-related disorders, there is some evidence to support the use of certain medications and of psychotherapeutic interventions. Relapse rates are high.

**Key Points**

- Motivational interviewing is a psychotherapeutic technique that can be used to target ambivalence and assess readiness for change in patients with stimulant-related disorders.
- Be sure to screen for use of other substances in patients who abuse stimulants.
- Use harm-reduction techniques.
- Optimize treatment of psychiatric comorbidities.

## References

1. Substance Abuse and Mental Health Services Administration. Key substance use and mental health indicators in the United States: Results from the 2018 National Survey on Drug Use and Health (HHS Publication No. PEP19-5068, NSDUH Series H-54). Rockville: Center for Behavioral Health Statistics and Quality, Substance Abuse and Mental Health Services Administration; 2019. Retrieved from https://www.samhsa.gov/data/.
2. Center for Behavioral Health Statistics and Quality. 2015 National Survey on drug use and health: detailed tables. Rockville: Substance Abuse and Mental Health Services Administration; 2016.
3. Degenhardt L, Chiu WT, Sampson N, Kessler RC, Anthony JC. Epidemiological patterns of extra-medical drug use in the United States: evidence from the national comorbidity survey replication, 2001–2003. Drug Alcohol Depend. 2007;90(2–3):210–23.
4. Anglin MD, Burke C, Perrochet B, Stamper E, Dawud-Noursi S. History of the methamphetamine problem. J Psychoactive Drugs. 2000;32(2):137–41. https://doi.org/10.1080/02791072.2000.10400221. PMID: 10908000.
5. Durell TM, Kroutil LA, Crits-Christoph P, Barchha N, Van Brunt DL. Prevalence of nonmedical methamphetamine use in the United States. Subst Abuse Treat Prev Policy. 2008;3:19. https://doi.org/10.1186/1747-597X-3-19. PMID: 18655714; PMCID: PMC2515829.
6. Rawson RA, Anglin MD, Ling W. Will the methamphetamine problem go away? J Addict Dis. 2002;21(1):5–19. https://doi.org/10.1300/j069v21n01_02. PMID: 11831500.
7. Harris D, Batki SL. Stimulant psychosis: symptom profile and acute clinical course. Am J Addict. 2000;9(1):28–37. https://doi.org/10.1080/10550490050172209. PMID: 10914291.
8. Grant KM, LeVan TD, Wells SM, et al. Methamphetamine-associated psychosis. J Neuroimmune Pharmacol. 2012;7(1):113–39. https://doi.org/10.1007/s11481-011-9288-1.
9. Colfax GN, Santos GM, Das M, Santos DM, Matheson T, Gasper J, Shoptaw S, Vittinghoff E. Mirtazapine to reduce methamphetamine use: a randomized controlled trial. Arch Gen Psychiatry. 2011;68(11):1168–75. https://doi.org/10.1001/archgenpsychiatry.2011.124. PMID: 22065532; PMCID: PMC3437988.
10. Coffin PO, Santos GM, Hern J, Vittinghoff E, Walker JE, Matheson T, Santos D, Colfax G, Batki SL. Effects of mirtazapine for methamphetamine use disorder among cisgender men and transgender women who have sex with men: a placebo-controlled randomized clinical trial. JAMA Psychiat. 2020;77(3):246–55. https://doi.org/10.1001/jamapsychiatry.2019.3655. PMID: 31825466; PMCID: PMC6990973.
11. Trivedi MH, Walker R, Ling W, Dela Cruz A, Sharma G, Carmody T, Ghitza UE, Wahle A, Kim M, Shores-Wilson K, Sparenborg S, Coffin P, Schmitz J, Wiest K, Bart G, Sonne SC, Wakhlu S, Rush AJ, Nunes EV, Shoptaw S. Bupropion and naltrexone in methamphetamine use disorder. N Engl J Med. 2021;384(2):140–53. https://doi.org/10.1056/NEJMoa2020214. PMID: 33497547.

12. Levin FR, Mariani JJ, Pavlicova M, Choi CJ, Mahony AL, Brooks DJ, Bisaga A, Dakwar E, Carpenter KM, Naqvi N, Nunes EV, Kampman K. Extended release mixed amphetamine salts and topiramate for cocaine dependence: a randomized clinical replication trial with frequent users. Drug Alcohol Depend. 2020;206:107700. https://doi.org/10.1016/j.drugalcdep.2019.107700. PMID: 31753736; PMCID: PMC6980777.
13. Crits-Christoph P, Siqueland L, Blaine J, Frank A, Luborsky L, Onken LS, Muenz LR, Thase ME, Weiss RD, Gastfriend DR, Woody GE, Barber JP, Butler SF, Daley D, Salloum I, Bishop S, Najavits LM, Lis J, Mercer D, Griffin ML, Moras K, Beck AT. Psychosocial treatments for cocaine dependence: national institute on drug abuse collaborative cocaine treatment study. Arch Gen Psychiatry. 1999;56(6):493–502. https://doi.org/10.1001/archpsyc.56.6.493. PMID: 10359461.
14. Maude-Griffin PM, Hohenstein JM, Humfleet GL, Reilly PM, Tusel DJ, Hall SM. Superior efficacy of cognitive-behavioral therapy for urban crack cocaine abusers: main and matching effects. J Consult Clin Psychol. 1998;66(5):832–7. https://doi.org/10.1037//0022-006x.66.5.832. PMID: 9803702.
15. Alammehrjerdi Z, Briggs NE, Biglarian A, Mokri A, Dolan K. A randomized controlled trial of brief cognitive behavioral therapy for regular methamphetamine use in methadone treatment. J Psychoactive Drugs. 2019;51(3):280–9. https://doi.org/10.1080/02791072.2019.1578445. PMID: 30835643.
16. Carroll KM, Onken LS. Behavioral therapies for drug abuse. Am J Psychiatry. 2005;162(8):1452–60. https://doi.org/10.1176/appi.ajp.162.8.1452. PMID: 16055766; PMCID: PMC3633201.
17. Lussier JP, Heil SH, Mongeon JA, Badger GJ, Higgins ST. A meta-analysis of voucher-based reinforcement therapy for substance use disorders. Addiction. 2006;101(2):192–203. https://doi.org/10.1111/j.1360-0443.2006.01311.x. PMID: 16445548.
18. Wang D, Zhou C, Zhao M, Wu X, Chang YK. Dose-response relationships between exercise intensity, cravings, and inhibitory control in methamphetamine dependence: an ERPs study. Drug Alcohol Depend. 2016;161:331–9. https://doi.org/10.1016/j.drugalcdep.2016.02.023. PMID: 26946990.
19. Brecht ML, Herbeck D. Time to relapse following treatment for methamphetamine use: a long-term perspective on patterns and predictors. Drug Alcohol Depend. 2014;139:18–25. https://doi.org/10.1016/j.drugalcdep.2014.02.702. PMID: 24685563; PMCID: PMC4550209.
20. Akindipe T, Wilson D, Stein DJ. Psychiatric disorders in individuals with methamphetamine dependence: prevalence and risk factors. Metab Brain Dis. 2014;29(2):351–7. https://doi.org/10.1007/s11011-014-9496-5. PMID: 24532047.
21. McKetin R, Kothe A, Baker AL, Lee NK, Ross J, Lubman DI. Predicting abstinence from methamphetamine use after residential rehabilitation: findings from the methamphetamine treatment evaluation study. Drug Alcohol Rev. 2018;37(1):70–8. https://doi.org/10.1111/dar.12528. PMID: 28421682.
22. Marlatt GA, Gordon JR. Relapse prevention: maintenance strategies in the treatment of addictive behaviors. New York: Guilford Press; 1985.
23. Carroll KM. A cognitive-behavioral approach: treating cocaine addiction. Rockville: National Institute on Drug Abuse; 1998.
24. Miller WR, Rollnick S. Motivational interviewing: helping people change. New York: Guilford Press; 2013.

# Nicotine Dependence and Tobacco Use Disorder Treatment

# 10

Noel Carrillo

According to the 2013–2014 National Adult Tobacco Survey (NATS), the prevalence of tobacco use in the United States during that time was 21.3% of adults age 18 and over [1]. About 17% of US adults consumed tobacco via cigarette smoking, which delivers a high amount of nicotine to the brain and the rest of the body [11]. Even though the prevalence of tobacco use and smoking has decreased compared to prior decades, millions of people who are actively smoking will eventually develop medical complications as a result of it. More recently, electronic cigarettes or e-cigarettes have skyrocketed in popularity, introducing a new vehicle for nicotine addiction, raising the specter of a reversal in decades-long efforts to reduce nicotine use, and creating a host of uncertain health effects for users given the paucity of available longitudinal evidence. In an effort to combat tobacco and nicotine addiction, many pharmacological treatments have been developed to treat tobacco use disorder and help facilitate smoking cessation. In this chapter, we will discuss the current treatment options available for tobacco use disorder and smoking cessation by incorporating clinical vignettes and highlighting research data that supports these treatments.

Aside from cigarette smoking, tobacco and nicotine can come in various other forms including cigars, pipes, water pipes (hookah), electronic cigarettes (e-cigs), and formulations developed for chewing, dipping, or snuffing [18]. However, smoking still remains the most popular method of nicotine consumption at this time. E-cigarettes and vaping have rapidly gained popularity since their appearance on the market more than a decade ago. According to the 2011–2018 National Youth Tobacco Survey (NYTS), e-cigarette use increased among high school students from 1.5% in 2011 to 20.8% in 2018 [4]. E-cigarettes are also regularly used as a smoking cessation tool, with some emerging evidence confirming that this can lead to prolonged abstinence from cigarettes for some [15]. Despite the rise in

N. Carrillo (✉)
PGY-3 Psychiatry Resident, New York Presbyterian/Weill Cornell, New York, NY, USA
e-mail: noc9036@nyp.org



J. D. Avery, D. Hankins (eds.), *Addiction Medicine*, Psychiatry Update 2,
https://doi.org/10.1007/978-3-030-86430-9_10

e-cigarettes' popularity and popular conceptions of vaping as a harm reduction strategy, health and safety data remain limited. E-cigarettes create known exposure to a number of other toxic compounds [19].

Regardless of the formulation, all tobacco-related products have nicotine, which is a naturally produced alkaloid found in the tobacco plant that acts as an agonist in the nicotinic cholinergic receptors of the autonomic ganglia and other areas of the central nervous system [18]. The effects of nicotine are dose-dependent and mediated by the release of several neurotransmitters including acetylcholine, beta-endorphins, dopamine, norepinephrine, serotonin, and adrenocorticotropic hormone (ACTH). Stimulant effects of nicotine can include both vascular effects – such as peripheral vasoconstriction, hypertension, tachycardia, and increased cardiac output – and cognitive effects including increased alertness and insomnia. Nicotine also produces depressant effects, such as muscle relaxation and anxiety reduction. Withdrawal symptoms of nicotine include anxiety, poor concentration, irritability, and cravings for tobacco.

In addition to its short-term effects, nicotine has long-term effects associated with poor health outcomes, related to its delivery by tobacco products [18, 21]. About 400,000 people in the United States die prematurely as a result of smoking, which accounts for about one of every five deaths in the United States. Free radicals found in cigarettes and other tobacco products cause oxidative stress, inflammation, and DNA damage to the human body across multiple organ systems. The most common types of cancer associated with smoking include lung, head, neck, gastrointestinal, and cervical malignancies. Smoking also causes cardiovascular conditions including coronary artery disease, stroke, aortic aneurysms, and peripheral arterial disease, prompted by chemical products found in cigarettes that cause endothelial dysfunction, changes in lipid metabolism, increased myocardial oxygen demand, and prothrombic effects. Lung diseases, such as chronic obstructive pulmonary disease (COPD), are also commonly associated with smoking. When smoke enters the lungs, it causes inflammation, cilia destruction, and mucous gland hyperplasia resulting in pulmonary pathology. The reproductive system is also affected by smoking in both men and women. In pregnant women, smoking can lead to low birth weight, premature birth, ectopic pregnancy, teratogenic effects, and sudden infant death syndrome, while in men it causes erectile dysfunction. Additional effects from smoking include impaired immune functioning, increased infection risk, peptic ulcers, bone fractures, and diabetes-related complications.

The prevalence of tobacco use differs among various subgroups, reflecting both historical consumption patterns and socioeconomic and racial disparities. In 2015, the prevalence of cigarette smoking was 16.7% in men and 13.6% in women; decades ago many more men than women smoked, but this gap by sex has been gradually closing [14]. Smoking rates also differ by race, with American Indian/Alaska Natives having the highest prevalence of 21.9% and Asians having the lowest at 7.0%. Increased rates of smoking have been consistently noted in communities with lower incomes, lower education levels, and higher unemployment, among many other socioeconomic correlates [10]. Those with mental illness or other substance use disorders have higher rates of cigarette smoking compared to the general population.

Due to addictive properties of nicotine, many individuals who smoke or consume tobacco, eventually develop tobacco use disorder. According to [5], in order to meet criteria for tobacco use disorder, a person must have a problematic pattern of tobacco use that leads to clinical impairment or distress within a 12-month period. The person must meet at least two criteria that are listed under that definition. Please see Table 10.1 for criteria listed by the DSM-5.

In terms of treatment, there are both pharmacologic and non-pharmacologic approaches to tobacco use disorder and smoking cessation. Most of the discussion of the rest of this chapter will focus on the evidence-based medication treatments currently available, which include nicotine replacement therapy (NRT), varenicline (also known as Chantix), and bupropion (also known as Wellbutrin). Please see Table 10.2 for a list of the medications as well as common doses for smoking cessation [21]. The following clinical cases will illustrate practical approaches to using these medications.

**Table 10.1** DSM-5 criteria for tobacco use disorder

| |
|---|
| A. A problematic pattern of tobacco use leading to clinically significant impairment or distress, as manifested by at least two of the following, occurring within a 12-month period: |
| 1. Tobacco is often taken in larger amounts or over a longer period than was intended |
| 2. There is a persistent desire or unsuccessful efforts to cut down or control tobacco use |
| 3. A great deal of time is spent in activities necessary to obtain or use tobacco |
| 4. Craving, or a strong desire or urge to use tobacco |
| 5. Recurrent tobacco use resulting in a failure to fulfill major role obligations at work, school, or home |
| 6. Continued tobacco use despite having persistent or recurrent social or interpersonal problems caused or exacerbated by the effects of tobacco (e.g., arguments with others about tobacco use) |
| 7. Important social, occupational, or recreational activities are given up or reduced because of tobacco use |
| 8. Recurrent tobacco use in situations in which it is physically hazardous (e.g., smoking in bed) |
| 9. Tobacco use is continued despite knowledge of having a persistent or recurrent physical or psychological problem that is likely to have been caused or exacerbated by tobacco |
| 10. Tolerance, as defined by either of the following:<br>(a). A need for markedly increased amounts of tobacco to achieve the desired effect<br>(b) A markedly diminished effect with continued use of the same amount of tobacco |
| 11. Withdrawal, as manifested by either of the following:<br>(a) The characteristic withdrawal syndrome for tobacco (refer to Criteria A and B of the criteria set for tobacco withdrawal)<br>(b) Tobacco (or a closely related substance, such as nicotine) is taken to relieve or avoid withdrawal symptoms |

**Table 10.2** Psychopharmacology of tobacco use disorders and dosing

| Name of medication | Dosing |
|---|---|
| Varenicline (Chantix) | Dosing: 0.5 mg, 1 mg<br>Frequency: 0.5 mg daily for days 1–3, then twice a day for days 4–7, then 1 mg twice a day starting day 8 and thereafter<br>Note: start 1 week before quit date |
| Bupropion (Wellbutrin, Zyban) | Dosing: 150 mg of the sustained-release formulation<br>Frequency: daily for days 1–3, then twice a day starting day 4 and thereafter<br>Note: start 1 week before quit date |
| Nicotine replacement therapies | Transdermal patch:<br>Doses: 7 mg, 14 mg, 21 mg<br>Frequency: every 24 hours<br>gum:<br>Doses: 2 mg, 4 mg<br>Frequency: every 1–2 h<br>Lozenge:<br>Doses: 2 mg, 4 mg<br>Frequency: every 1–2 h<br>Sublingual tablet:<br>Doses: 2 mg, 4 mg<br>Frequency: every 1–2 h<br>Inhalation:<br>Doses: 1 cartridge<br>Frequency: continuously every 20 minutes but no more than 16 cartridges/day<br>Nasal spray:<br>Doses: 1 mg per dose (2 sprays)<br>Frequency: 1–2 doses per hour |

## Clinical Cases

Dr. Ramos recently completed residency in psychiatry and started an addiction psychiatry fellowship. During her first week as a fellow, she discusses three cases with her attending related to tobacco use disorder and her proposed treatments. Her first case, Jonathan, is a 39-year-old man with a history of anxiety, who has never seen a therapist before and has never taken medication in the past because of "trouble swallowing pills." Jonathan reports that he has been smoking about two packs a day and is interested in quitting. He is willing to try "anything," including therapy and medication.

Her next case is Xavier, a 65-year-old-man with a history of depression, previously on SSRIs but stopped due to sexual side effects. Lately he has been feeling more depressed with low energy, increased sleep, and weight gain. He attributes his low mood to the fact that he has failed to quit smoking in the past but is thinking of attempting to quit again. He has been smoking a pack of cigarettes a day almost every day for the last 20 years. He reports wanting to quit because recently he was diagnosed with coronary artery disease and hypertension. Xavier is now interested in medication that can help him in both smoking cessation and his depression.

Dr. Ramos's final patient is Nataly, a 20-year-old woman with a history of an eating disorder in the past and seizures. She began smoking half a pack of cigarettes a day two years ago when she turned 18 and started college. She has attempted to quit in the past by using nicotine gum and patch, but her attempts were unsuccessful. Lately, she has been vaping and using e-cigarettes, which help to reduce her cravings but at times she continues to smoke cigarettes, especially during her final examinations. Nataly is interested in trying another medication to help her quit before next month when school starts again.

## Discussion

Dr. Ramos's patients are presenting with nicotine dependence and would benefit from treatment. Each of the available treatments has strengths and weaknesses, detailed in Table 10.3 [21, 24]. For each of these cases, there are specific factors in the history and presentation of these patients that might persuade a provider to choose one medication over another. For the rest of the chapter, we will discuss the current treatments available for tobacco use disorder and why Dr. Ramos might choose that particular treatment over the others.

## Non-pharmacological Intervention

In our first case, Jonathan is interested in both therapy and medication. After a person stops smoking, there are many psychological factors that can lead someone to relapse including intermittent negative thoughts and emotions, multiple urges to smoke, decreased motivation, and self-efficacy about quitting. Therefore, there are a variety of interventions that have been shown to be effective in helping to prevent relapse of smoking and tobacco use [21]. Some of these non-pharmaceutical interventions include cognitive behavioral therapy (CBT), motivational interviewing, and acceptance and commitment therapy. These therapies can be individual or group based and vary in intensity. Nicotine Anonymous is another option, with hundreds of 12-step meetings available worldwide. They can also vary by mode of delivery, which can include delivery by a clinician, counselor, telephone, or computer. Most research supports their efficacy in increasing smoking cessation rates, but data comparing each of these modes is limited. However, data does show that effectiveness is dose-responsive, so higher amounts of exposure to these behavioral strategies yield longer periods of sustained cessation.

## Nicotine Replacement Treatment

Another option for Jonathan is nicotine replacement therapy (NRT), which helps by reducing nicotine cravings in those that smoke or use tobacco. NRT comes in five forms including a transdermal patch, gum, lozenge, nasal spray, and inhaler [22].

**Table 10.3** Comparison of different treatments in smoking cessation

| Intervention | Advantages | Disadvantages |
|---|---|---|
| Psychosocial treatment only (brief provider interventions, individual psychological interventions, telephone support, Nicotine Anonymous, etc.) | Can address psychological factors and motivation to quit<br>Brief interventions still effective<br>Maximizes social support to help patient quit<br>More effective than self-help | Does not address biological dependence, cravings, or withdrawal symptoms<br>Less intensive interventions shown to be less effective |
| Nicotine replacement therapy | Low cost<br>Different formulations chosen based on patient preference<br>Has both short-acting and long-acting forms, which can help with withdrawal and craving symptoms<br>Mimics hand to mouth ritual<br>Few side effects | More frequent dosing for short-acting forms<br>Irritation of the skin, mouth, or nose depending on formulation used<br>Less effective than varenicline |
| Bupropion | Simple twice a day dosing<br>No weight gain<br>Can help with depression<br>Can be combined with NRT | Adverse effects can include insomnia, anxiety, dry mouth<br>Contraindicated in patients with history of eating disorder or seizures or concurrent use of monoamine oxidase inhibitors (MAOIs)<br>Must monitor neuropsychiatric symptoms<br>Less effective than varenicline |
| Varenicline | Simple dosing of twice a day<br>Different mechanism of action for patient who have failed other treatments<br>Most effective treatment | Adverse effects include nausea, vomiting, constipation, sleep disturbances<br>Must monitor neuropsychiatric symptoms<br>Limited data suggests cardiovascular effects |

This is particularly convenient for someone like Jonathan, who doesn't like "swallowing pills." These formulations work by providing nicotine without the other hazardous chemicals found in cigarettes or tobacco. NRT provides lower doses of nicotine that normally last longer than nicotine found in cigarettes or tobacco. The nicotine patch provides the longest release of nicotine [22].

All forms of NRT increase rate of quitting by 50–60%, and efficacy is comparable among the different formulations [9]. However, based on research, combining the long-acting nicotine patch with a short-acting form is more effective than a single NRT agent. A Cochrane meta-analysis found that this combined approach made quitting 15–36% more likely. [16]. Therefore, Dr. Ramos may want to prescribe Jonathan a long-acting patch with a short-acting form, such as nicotine gum, in hopes that this will be more effective in helping Jonathan quit smoking.

In general, NRT has a low side effect profile, including heart palpitations and chest pains, nausea and vomiting, insomnia, as well as irritation of the mouth and skin depending on route of administration [17]. Therefore, NRT is the safest pharmacological treatment to prescribe, particularly since most individuals prescribed NRT will already be habituated to these physiologic effects of nicotine.

## Bupropion

Bupropion is an effective medication for smoking cessation and tobacco use disorder that is also a treatment for depression [8]. Therefore, Xavier might benefit from this medication as it would help both with his tobacco use disorder and his mood. The mechanism of this drug related to smoking cessation is not totally clear [23]. When nicotine crosses the blood-brain barrier, it causes a release of dopamine into the synaptic cleft of the dopaminergic, pleasure-seeking pathways of the brain. Similarly, bupropion blocks the reuptake of dopamine. Additionally, it is thought that dopamine deficiency in the nucleus accumbens leads to nicotine withdrawal when smoking is stopped. Therefore, bupropion might increase dopamine in the nucleus accumbens, which leads to attenuation of nicotine withdrawal symptoms. Bupropion is also a noncompetitive blocker of the postsynaptic acetylcholine nicotine receptor, which stops the reinforcing effect of nicotine use [23].

Bupropion appears to be an effective treatment of tobacco use disorder. A meta-analysis of 65 RCTs found that bupropion as a monotherapy significantly increased long-term cessation of 6 months or greater (RR = 1.62; 95% CI, 1.49–1.76) relative to placebo, which was comparable to NRT (RR = 0.96; 95% CI, 0.85–1.09) [13]. A Cochrane meta-analysis also found that both bupropion and NRT are comparable in efficacy [3].

Bupropion's most common side effects include headache, insomnia, dry mouth, and agitation [12]. However, one of the most notable adverse effects is seizures [12]. The risk of seizures depends both on dose and on preparation. The higher the dose, the higher the risk of developing seizures. Additionally, the sustained-release formulation has a lower risk of seizures compared to the immediate-release formulation. Therefore, seizure disorder is a major contraindication to use, as well as any other factors that predispose someone to seizures including discontinuation of alcohol or sedatives, arteriovenous malformations, severe headache injury, stroke, brain tumor, or any other significant central nervous system disease. Bupropion should also not be used in someone with a history of an eating disorder or bipolar disorder or who is on monoamine oxidase inhibitors [12]. Therefore bupropion would not be an appropriate medication to use in someone like Nataly, who has a history of an eating disorder and seizures.

The FDA requires all antidepressants to carry a boxed warning that antidepressants can increase risk of suicide in those under 25 years of age, including bupropion. However, suicidal behavior is less of a concern in smoking cessation. In

December 2016, data from a large clinical trial convinced the FDA that serious mood and suicidal behaviors were not as severe as previously thought of and the FDA removed the black box warning for smoking cessation [19]. The report still advises to use with caution and to monitor behavioral symptoms, especially in patients with co-occurring mood or psychotic disorders.

## Varenicline

Another medication option for tobacco use disorder is varenicline, which may be an ideal option for Nataly. This drug works as a partial agonist of the alpha-4-beta-2 nicotinic acetylcholine receptor subtype (nACh) [20]. When the drug attaches to the receptor, it produces less effect of dopamine release than it would with nicotine. This leads to decreased nicotine addiction, and it also decreases the cravings and withdrawal syndrome associated with cessation of tobacco use.

Varenicline appears to be the most effective option for tobacco use disorder. A study assessing the effectiveness of varenicline in smokers who had no intention to quit in the next 30 days found that 32.1% of smokers were biochemically confirmed to have been continuously abstinent by weeks 15–24 after starting varenicline [6]. On the other hand, the placebo group only had an abstinence of 6.9% during that time period. Additionally, by weeks 21–52 after initiation of the trial, 27% of the varenicline group remained abstinent, compared to only 9% in the placebo group. A Cochrane review also found that varenicline is more effective than either NRT or bupropion [3]. The odds ratio of effectiveness compared to placebo was 1.84 (95% CI of 1.71–1.99) for NRT, 1.82 (95% CI 1.60–2.06) for bupropion, and 2.88 (95% CI 2.40–3.47) for varenicline.

The most common side effect of varenicline is nausea, which is seen in almost 30% of people taking it [7]. Other less common side effects include headache, insomnia, vivid dreams, constipation, and other gastrointestinal symptoms. In 2009, the US FDA required that varenicline carries a boxed warning that the drug should be stopped if there were any changes in behavior. This was done in response to post-marketing reports carried out by the FDA that found increased suicidality risk and suicidal behavior among people using varenicline for smoking cessation. However, many systematic reviews have been conducted that have found no increased suicide risk or neuropsychiatric side effects. In 2016, the FDA removed the black box warning as it did for bupropion, but the FDA continues to recommend monitoring patients for these side effects [19]. In June 2011, the US FDA also issued a safety announcement about varenicline potentially causing a small increase of cardiovascular adverse events in people with cardiovascular disease. This was based on a review that showed increased risk of cardiovascular events in people using varenicline compared to placebo. However, multiple reviews and meta-analyses afterward have found no increase in cardiovascular events associated with varenicline use [6]. Given that Xavier already has history of cardiovascular disease, it may be prudent to try a medication other than varenicline given possible risk of cardiovascular events.

A number of studies have also looked at combination therapies combining varenicline with other smoking cessation medications [2]. A study showed higher continuous abstinence in those who combined varenicline with a 15 mg nicotine patch compared to those who were on varenicline alone. However, another study found no difference. In another study that looked at varenicline plus bupropion, there were no differences found between the two groups in terms of abstinence. However, a subgroup analysis found significantly higher rates of abstinence in those who smoked more than 20 cigarettes per day [2]. Therefore, combining varenicline with bupropion might be another option for some patients.

## Conclusion

Although prevalence rates for tobacco use disorder are decreasing around the world, millions of people worldwide continue to consume tobacco and are at increased risk of serious illness and death as a result of it. Providers must continue to discuss tobacco and nicotine use with their patients, keeping in mind the variety of potential nicotine delivery methods and the recent surge in popularity of e-cigarettes. A treatment plan including psychosocial and/or pharmacologic interventions for tobacco use disorder can be individually tailored to a patient's preferences and relevant additional information in the history that might make certain options a better fit than others.

### Key Points

- Nicotine use remains a major cause of morbidity and mortality around the world, primarily because of its delivery through harmful tobacco products.
- Tobacco use disorder is a DSM-5 diagnosis that can be made based on an individual's pattern of problematic tobacco use.
- Both behavioral and pharmacological interventions on their own, or in combination, can be used to treat tobacco use disorder.
- Currently, there are three medication options to help with smoking cessation: nicotine replacement therapy, bupropion, and varenicline.
- The differences in these medications' required frequency, side effect profiles, contraindications, and effectiveness should all be considered when working with a patient to craft a plan for nicotine cessation.

## References

1. Agaku IT, King BA, Husten CG, Bunnell R, Ambrose BK, Hu SS, Holder-Hayes E, Day HR, Centers for Disease Control and Prevention (CDC). Tobacco product use among adults–United States, 2012–2013. MMWR Morb Mortal Wkly Rep. 2014;63(25):542–7. Erratum in: MMWR Morb Mortal Wkly Rep. 2014 Jul 4;63(26):576. PMID: 24964880; PMCID: PMC5779380.

2. Burke MV, Hays JT, Ebbert JO. Varenicline for smoking cessation: a narrative review of efficacy, adverse effects, use in at-risk populations, and adherence. Patient Prefer Adherence. 2016;10:435–41. https://doi.org/10.2147/PPA.S83469. PMID: 27099479; PMCID: PMC4824380.
3. Cahill K, Stevens S, Perera R, Lancaster T. Pharmacological interventions for smoking cessation: an overview and network meta-analysis. Cochrane Database Syst Rev 2013;(5):CD009329. doi: https://doi.org/10.1002/14651858.CD009329.pub2. PMID: 23728690.
4. Cullen KA, Ambrose BK, Gentzke AS, Apelberg BJ, Jamal A, King BA. Notes from the field: use of electronic cigrettes and any tobacco product among middle and high school student – United States, 2011–2018. MMWR Morb Mortal Wkly Rep. 2018;67:1276–7.
5. DSM-V. Diagnostic and statistical manual of mental disorders: DSM-5. 5th ed. American Psychiatric Association; 2013.
6. Ebbert JO, Hughes JR, West RJ, Rennard SI, Russ C, McRae TD, Treadow J, Yu CR, Dutro MP, Park PW. Effect of varenicline on smoking cessation through smoking reduction: a randomized clinical trial. JAMA. 2015;313(7):687–94. https://doi.org/10.1001/jama.2015.280. PMID: 25688780; PMCID: PMC4883651.
7. Ebbert JO, Wyatt KD, Hays JT, Klee EW, Hurt RD. Varenicline for smoking cessation: efficacy, safety, and treatment recommendations. Patient Prefer Adherence. 2010;4:355–62. https://doi.org/10.2147/ppa.s10620. PMID: 21049087; PMCID: PMC2962400.
8. Fava M, Rush AJ, Thase ME, Clayton A, Stahl SM, Pradko JF, Johnston JA. 15 years of clinical experience with bupropion HCl: from bupropion to bupropion SR to bupropion XL. Prim care companion. J Clin Psychiatry. 2005;7(3):106–13. https://doi.org/10.4088/pcc.v07n0305. PMID: 16027765; PMCID: PMC1163271.
9. Hartmann-Boyce J, Chepkin SC, Ye W, Bullen C, Lancaster T. Nicotine replacement therapy versus control for smoking cessation. Cochrane Database Syst Rev. 2018;5(5):CD000146. https://doi.org/10.1002/14651858.CD000146.pub5. PMID: 29852054; PMCID: PMC6353172.
10. Hiscock R, Bauld L, Amos A, Fidler JA, Munafò M. Socioeconomic status and smoking: a review. Ann N Y Acad Sci. 2012;1248(1):107–23.
11. Hu SS, Neff L, Agaku IT, Cox S, Day HR, Holder-Hayes E, King BA. Tobacco product use among adults – United States, 2013–2014. MMWR Morb Mortal Wkly Rep. 2016;65(27):685–91. https://doi.org/10.15585/mmwr.mm6527a1. PMID: 27416365.
12. Huecker MR, Smiley A, Saadabadi A. Bupropion. Treasure Island: StatPearls Publishing; 2020. PMID: 29262173.
13. Hughes JR, Stead LF, Hartmann-Boyce J, Cahill K, Lancaster T. Antidepressants for smoking cessation. Cochrane Database Syst Rev. 2014;2014(1):CD000031. https://doi.org/10.1002/14651858.CD000031.pub4. Update in: Cochrane Database Syst Rev. 2020 Apr 22;4:CD000031. PMID: 24402784; PMCID: PMC7027688
14. Jamal A, King BA, Neff LJ, Whitmill J, Babb SD, Graffunder CM. Current cigarette smoking among adults—United States, 2005–2015. Morb Mortal Wkly Rep. 2016;65:1205–11. https://doi.org/10.15585/mmwr.mm6544a2.
15. Kalkhoran S, Chang Y, Rigotti NA. Electronic cigarette use and cigarette abstinence over 2 years among U.S. smokers in the population assessment of tobacco and health study. Nicotine Tob Res. 2020;22(5):728–33. https://doi.org/10.1093/ntr/ntz114.
16. Lindson N, Chepkin SC, Ye W, Fanshawe TR, Bullen C, Hartmann-Boyce J. Different doses, durations and modes of delivery of nicotine replacement therapy for smoking cessation. Cochrane Database Syst Rev. 2019;4(4):CD013308. https://doi.org/10.1002/14651858.CD013308. PMID: 30997928; PMCID: PMC6470854.
17. Mills EJ, Wu P, Lockhart I, Wilson K, Ebbert JO. Adverse events associated with nicotine replacement therapy (NRT) for smoking cessation. A systematic review and meta-analysis of one hundred and twenty studies involving 177,390 individuals. Tob Induc Dis. 2010;8(1):8. https://doi.org/10.1186/1617-9625-8-8. PMID: 20626883; PMCID: PMC2917405.
18. Onor IO, Stirling DL, Williams SR, Bediako D, Borghol A, Harris MB, Darensburg TB, Clay SD, Okpechi SC, Sarpong DF. Clinical effects of cigarette smoking: epidemiologic impact

and review of pharmacotherapy options. Int J Environ Res Public Health. 2017;14(10):1147. https://doi.org/10.3390/ijerph14101147. PMID: 28956852; PMCID: PMC5664648.
19. Safety Alerts for Human Medical Products – Chantix (varenicline) and Zyban (bupropion): Drug safety communication – mental health side effects revised. U.S. food and drug administration (FDA). Archived from the original on 20 December 2016. Retrieved 20 December 2016.
20. Singh D, Saadabadi A. Varenicline. Treasure Island: StatPearls Publishing; 2020.
21. United States Public Health Service Office of the Surgeon General; National Center for Chronic Disease Prevention and Health Promotion (US) Office on Smoking and Health. Smoking cessation: a report of the surgeon general. Washington, DC: US Department of Health and Human Services; 2020. Chapter 6, Interventions for Smoking Cessation and Treatments for Nicotine Dependence.
22. Wadgave U, Nagesh L. Nicotine replacement therapy: an overview. Int J Health Sci (Qassim). 2016;10(3):425–35. PMID: 27610066; PMCID: PMC5003586.
23. Wilkes S. The use of bupropion SR in cigarette smoking cessation. Int J Chron Obstruct Pulmon Dis. 2008;3(1):45–53. https://doi.org/10.2147/copd.s1121. PMID: 18488428; PMCID: PMC2528204.
24. Ziedonis D, Das S, Larkin C. Tobacco use disorder and treatment: new challenges and opportunities. Dialogues Clin Neurosci. 2017;19(3):271–80. https://doi.org/10.31887/DCNS.2017.19.3/dziedonis. PMID: 29302224; PMCID: PMC5741110.

# Behavioral Addictions

# 11

Daniel Sugrue

In the past, addiction mainly referred to the recurrent compulsive and maladaptive use of alcohol or other substances with associated functional impairment. However, a growing body of research has shown significant overlap between substance use disorders (SUDs) and the compulsive engagement of problematic behaviors. These behaviors include gambling, Internet gaming, sexual behavior, eating, and shopping, among others. Given this overlap, some have come to classify the recurrent dysfunctional engagement of these behaviors as behavioral addictions. However, debate about whether these behaviors should be recognized as actual addictive disorders continues to this day [1]. Several behaviors have been shown to have significant overlap with SUDs and have been described using the addiction model. These include gambling disorder, Internet gaming disorder, and hypersexual disorder. This chapter will focus on these three conditions and discuss their clinical characteristics, including diagnostic criteria and prevalent psychiatric comorbidities, as well as their potential treatment options.

Gambling disorder is the only non-substance-related disorder found in the "Substance Related and Addictive Disorders" section in the Fifth Edition of the *Diagnostic and Statistical Manual of Mental Disorders* (DSM-5). This categorization is different from the previous DSM-IV, in which the American Psychiatric Association (APA) had recognized disordered gambling, previously known as pathological gambling, as an impulse-control disorder. This alteration not only reinforced the similarities between gambling disorder and SUDs, but also supported the notion that maladaptive engagement of a behavior could be classified as an addictive disorder [1]. Similar to the APA, the World Health Organization (WHO) also recognized disordered gambling as an addictive disorder in the eleventh revision of the International Classification of Diseases (ICD-11) [2].

D. Sugrue (✉)
General Adult Psychiatry Resident, Weill Cornell Medical College, New York, NY, USA
e-mail: das2045@nyp.org



J. D. Avery, D. Hankins (eds.), *Addiction Medicine*, Psychiatry Update 2,
https://doi.org/10.1007/978-3-030-86430-9_11

According to the DSM-5, patients with gambling disorder may often be preoccupied with gambling, increase the amount of money they gamble to experience the same level of excitement, try to cover up their amount of gambling from others, gamble in response to stress or to recover previous losses, and rely on others financially to continue their gambling. Patients with the disorder may also experience negative mood states when not gambling, risk or lose relationships or career opportunities due to gambling, and have failed to quit gambling on numerous occasions. To meet a diagnosis of gambling disorder, one needs to exhibit at least four of the above symptoms in a 12-month period, and their behavior cannot be attributed to a manic episode [1, 2].

The lifetime prevalence of disordered gambling in the United States has been found to range from 0.4% to 0.6% and has been associated with reduced quality of life and significant patient distress. Patients with gambling disorder are more likely to experience bankruptcy, legal trouble, marital problems, and medical ailments such as cirrhosis and other forms of liver disease due to comorbid alcohol abuse. Indeed, disordered gambling has been associated with a high prevalence of comorbid SUDs as well as comorbid mood and anxiety disorders, personality disorders, and impulse control disorders. Between 17% and 24% of patients with gambling disorder have reported attempting suicide because of distress tied to their gambling. Despite the significant impairment associated with gambling disorder, however, only about 10% of individuals seek treatment, with their motivation being often tied to legal, financial, or interpersonal difficulties [2]. These clinical characteristics highlight the importance of screening patients with gambling disorder for comorbid psychiatric symptoms, as well as screening for symptoms of disordered gambling among patients seeking help for other psychiatric symptoms. In addition, physicians should keep in mind that patients with gambling disorder may also have other problematic behaviors, which are often linked, as in the case of gambling and Internet gaming [3].

Gaming, similar to gambling, was recognized by the WHO as an addictive behavior, which eventually included gaming disorder as a medical condition in the ICD-11. In the ICD-11, this disorder is characterized by excessive gaming that is difficult to control, persists despite negative consequences, and is associated with functional impairment over at least a year period [4]. The APA, on the other hand, categorized Internet gaming disorder in Section III of the DSM-5, which requires that further research be done before the condition can be officially recognized as a disorder. The proposed symptoms of Internet gaming disorder include a preoccupation with gaming, a loss of interest in other activities due to gaming, and an inability to stop gaming despite negative consequences. Patients with this condition may also try to cover up their amount of gaming from others, experience distress when not gaming, spend increasing amounts of time gaming to achieve the same level of excitement, game in response to stress, and jeopardize relationships or career opportunities due to gaming. In order to receive a diagnosis of Internet gaming disorder, one needs to exhibit at least five of these symptoms in a one-year period [5].

In the midst of the controversy over whether gaming ought to be considered an addictive behavior, an increasing number of studies have looked at the prevalence rates and clinical characteristics of Internet gaming disorder. Prevalence rates have been found to range between 1% and 10% in European and North American populations and 10% and 15% in East and Southeast Asian populations. Internet gaming disorder is more common among males and younger individuals and has been associated with increased social difficulties, physical aggression, and poor academic performance. The physical well-being of individuals has also been shown to be jeopardized in certain cases due to sleep disturbances and decreased food and fluid intake [6]. In addition, Internet gaming disorder has been associated with SUDs and other comorbid psychiatric disorders including mood, anxiety, and personality disorders [7]. Hence, similar to the approach to gambling disorder, providers should screen for these comorbid psychiatric symptoms in patients presenting with Internet gaming disorder symptoms, in addition to other associated problematic behaviors, such as hypersexual behavior.

Hypersexual disorder, a term that has been used interchangeably with hypersexuality, compulsive sexual behavior disorder, and sexual addiction, was proposed for addition to the DSM-5, with an addiction model framework. The proposed diagnostic criteria included recurrent sexual thoughts, urges, and behaviors that are difficult to control, often occur in response to negative mood states, take up excessive time, and impair an individual's functioning. In addition, the condition can include participation in sexual behaviors that endanger the safety of the patient or others. These behaviors may include cybersex, pornography use, masturbation, and sexual activity with multiple partners, among others. Furthermore, these symptoms cannot be attributed to mania, substance abuse, or drug side effects [8]. The APA ultimately did not recognize hypersexual disorder as an addictive disorder in the DSM-5, however, stating that more supporting evidence for its inclusion was needed. The WHO, meanwhile, categorized hypersexual behavior as an impulse-control disorder in the ICD-11, using the term compulsive sexual behavior disorder [8]. Despite the ongoing debate over its characterization, many clinicians recognize hypersexual disorder as an addictive disorder that can have detrimental effects on patients' careers, personal lives, and physical health [9]. The latter may be jeopardized due to increased risk for sexually transmitted diseases (STDs) and injury secondary to repeated intercourse. However, despite the associated impairment, hypersexual disorder often goes undiagnosed, and many patients don't seek treatment until well into their 30s (even though symptoms often start around 18 years of age) [9]. Also, similar to gambling disorder, the motivation to seek treatment is often tied to professional or legal troubles or related to their comorbid psychiatric disorders [9]. Given the delay among patients in seeking treatment for their hypersexual disorder, providers ought to screen for problematic sexual behaviors, in addition to others (i.e., gambling and gaming), in patients presenting with other psychiatric symptoms.

Gambling disorder, Internet gaming disorder, and hypersexual disorder often occur in individuals with other co-occurring disorders. These include SUDs, mood and anxiety disorders, impulse-control disorders, and personality disorders, among others. Table 11.1 highlights the prevalence rates of different psychiatric comorbidities among patients with these problematic behaviors, based on several epidemiological studies [9–11]. This association with other

**Table 11.1** Prevalence rates of comorbid psychiatric disorders in behavioral addictions

| Pathological gambling | Internet gaming disorder | Hypersexual disorder |
|---|---|---|
| Alcohol use disorder (73.2%) | Anxiety (92%) | Mood disorders (72%) |
| Personality disorder (60.8%) | Depression (89%) | Other addictive disorders (40–71%) |
| Nicotine dependence (60.4%) | Attention-Deficit/Hyperactivity Disorder (ADHD) (87%) | Anxiety disorders (38%) |
| Mood disorder (49.6%) | Social phobia/anxiety and obsessive compulsive symptoms (75%) | ADHD (17–19%) |
| Anxiety disorder (41.3%) | – | Personality disorders (17%) |
| Drug use disorder (38.1%) | – | Obsessive-Compulsive Disorder (OCD) (12–14%) |
| – | – | Impulse control disorders (5–6%) |

psychiatric disorders calls attention to the importance of obtaining a comprehensive history from patients to not only rule out other primary causes for their symptoms (i.e., mania, substance use), but also screen for comorbid psychiatric diagnoses to treat [2, 9].

An increasing number of studies have examined evidence-based treatments for gaming disorder, Internet gaming disorder, and hypersexual disorder that include pharmacologic and psychosocial interventions. When used in combination, these interventions have shown some promising results in improving patients' symptoms for these disorders. Furthermore, medications that have been able to improve these behavioral addictions have also been able to target comorbid psychiatric symptoms [2, 5, 9]. Treatment approaches are discussed later.

The following three clinical cases exemplify the benefit in screening patients for symptoms of both behavioral addictions and other psychiatric disorders to inform optimal treatment. In particular, a thorough assessment of these symptoms can inform a provider's medication selection to target both problematic behaviors and comorbid psychiatric symptoms.

## Clinical Cases

Dr. Jones is a psychiatry resident treating patients at his hospital's outpatient clinic. He is scheduled to conduct an initial evaluation of three patients who were referred to the clinic and develop individualized treatment plans for each case.

The first patient Dr. Jones interviews is Mr. F., a 57-year-old married man, employed as an attorney, with a family history notable for alcohol use disorder, not currently on any medications, who presents at the behest of his wife to request help in stopping gambling. Over the last year, he describes having gambled five nights out of the week at the casino near his home, which he has tried to hide from his wife and the rest of his family. He reports experiencing a persistent and intense urge to gamble, has lost nearly all of his savings from gambling this past year, and has had to borrow money from his brother to continue gambling. He has been unable to stop on his own, despite multiple attempts, and has come seeking help only after his wife threatened to divorce him if he did not seek counseling. On screening for substance use, Dr. Jones learns that Mr. F. has a history of binge drinking a six-pack of beer three nights out of the week for several decades, which has increased to six nights over the past year. He denies having received any treatment in the past to reduce his alcohol consumption but is open to considering options to help curb his drinking.

The second patient Dr. Jones evaluates is Ms. C., a 20-year-old woman, currently enrolled as a junior in college, with no significant psychiatric history, who was referred to the clinic by her academic advisor, who expressed concern about Ms. C.'s apparent low mood, loss of interest in activities, and associated decline in school performance over the past year. On interview, Ms. C. reports feeling depressed for the past 2 months with associated poor sleep, energy, and appetite and has had thoughts that life is not worth living. When asked about her interest in activities, she reports that she had previously enjoyed spending time with friends and participating in extracurricular activities, but that she gradually gave these up in favor of playing an online video game. Ms. C. reports having been introduced to the game a little over a year ago, which she initially played for one hour each day, but has since progressed to about nine hours a day. She reports heightened irritability and restlessness when not gaming and has kept the extent of her gaming hidden from her family. She reports, however, that her grades have suffered because of her gaming and is now at risk of academic probation. She reports having tried to quit gaming multiple times, but hasn't been successful. She now expresses interest in receiving treatment for both her mood symptoms and problematic gaming.

The third case of the day is Mr. R., a 31-year-old single man, currently employed as a consultant, with a history of generalized anxiety disorder, not on medications, who was referred to the clinic for mandated treatment after being caught masturbating to pornography at work. On interview, he expresses significant distress about his masturbatory habits over the past couple of years, which he describes as excessive. He reports experiencing the intense urge to masturbate throughout most of the day, finds this urge difficult to control, and often experiences the urge more often when under stress. When Dr. Jones asks about his anxiety, Mr. R. reports having felt anxious throughout his life, including constantly feeling "on edge." He also describes having difficulty making simple decisions, has trouble falling asleep most nights, and finds it difficult to concentrate. He reports being interested in receiving treatment to reduce his anxiety and the frequency he masturbates and uses pornography.

After seeing each patient, Dr. Jones reviews each case to prepare individualized treatment plans to include medications that target both the patients' problematic behaviors and comorbid psychiatric symptoms.

## Discussion of Clinical Cases

Dr. Jones' patients presented to the clinic for various reasons, and after a thorough assessment, he has elicited symptoms of behavioral addictions and some of their common psychiatric comorbidities. Each of these cases illustrates the significant interpersonal, academic, and professional problems that may occur with behavioral addictions and the resultant personal distress. Furthermore, they highlight that the problems associated with these conditions are often the reason patients are either referred to treatment or seek help on their own. Given the history he obtained on the interviews, Dr. Jones can now consider a combined approach with the available pharmacologic and psychosocial interventions to treat each patient. In particular, he can discuss medication options with the patients that target both their problematic behavior and comorbid psychiatric symptoms, as discussed in the following section.

## Gambling Disorder

Mr. F.'s description of his gambling behavior and the significant impairment this has caused in his life is consistent with a diagnosis of gambling disorder. His motivation to seek treatment due to the interpersonal difficulties his gambling disorder has caused with his wife is also one of the common reasons patients seek treatment for this disorder [2]. His alcohol use, combined with his family history, is also concerning for alcohol use disorder, and he would likely benefit from further discussion about his motivation to quit.

Currently, there is no medication approved by the US Food and Drug Administration (FDA) for the treatment of gambling disorder, but research has shown numerous medications to be effective, which is outlined in Table 11.2 [2]. With respect to this particular case, Dr. Jones may wish to consider an opioid receptor antagonist, such as naltrexone or nalmefene (the latter available in Europe), to treat both Mr. F.'s gambling disorder and alcohol use disorder [2]. An opioid antagonist may also lead to a better treatment outcome for this particular patient, in light of his intense gambling urges and family history of alcohol use disorder, both of

**Table 11.2** Preferred pharmacologic agents for gambling disorder based on psychiatric comorbidities

| Pharmacologic agent(s) | Psychiatric comorbidities targeted | |
|---|---|---|
| Opioid antagonists (naltrexone, nalmefene) | Alcohol use disorder | Opioid use disorder |
| Mood stabilizers (lithium and valproate) | Bipolar disorder or bipolar spectrum disorders | – |
| Glutamatergic agents (n-acetylcysteine) | Nicotine dependence | – |
| Selective serotonin reuptake inhibitors (escitalopram, paroxetine, fluvoxamine) | Mood disorders other than bipolar spectrum disorders | Anxiety disorders (generalized anxiety disorder, social anxiety disorder, etc.) |

which have been associated with positive outcomes for patients on these medications [1, 2].

In his approach to other patients, Dr. Jones may wish to consider other pharmacotherapy that has been studied in the treatment of gambling disorder. These include selective serotonin reuptake inhibitors (SSRIs), mood stabilizers, and glutamatergic agents. Escitalopram, an SSRI indicated for certain mood and anxiety disorders, may be an option for Dr. Jones to consider for patients with problematic gambling and comorbid mood and anxiety symptoms. However, the studies of SSRIs in treating gambling disorder, in particular paroxetine and fluvoxamine, have been equivocal. Meanwhile, in his approach to patients with comorbid bipolar disorder, mood stabilizers like lithium and valproate may be beneficial. Lastly, N-acetylcysteine (NAC), a glutamatergic agent, may be helpful for patients with gambling disorder and concurrent tobacco use, given that NAC has been shown to improve nicotine dependence and gambling disorder symptoms, when administered along with behavioral treatment [2].

In addition to pharmacotherapy, Dr. Jones should discuss the available psychosocial treatments for gambling disorder with Mr. F. These include Gamblers Anonymous, cognitive behavioral therapy (CBT), and motivational interviewing, all of which have been shown to effectively improve gambling disorder symptoms. Given the severity of Mr. F.'s gambling, he would likely benefit from a combination of Gamblers Anonymous and CBT, with the option of motivational interviewing. However, if he were not willing to commit to multiple modalities, Dr. Jones can assess his interest in engaging in at least one of them [2].

## Internet Gaming Disorder

Ms. C. was initially referred for treatment of her mood symptoms, which were thought to be associated with her decline in academic performance. However upon further assessment, Dr. Jones elicited information about the negative impact her problematic gaming behaviors has had, which dates back starting before her depressive symptoms. After obtaining a thorough history, he suspects a diagnosis of Internet gaming disorder with comorbid major depression, and her interest in receiving treatment gives Dr. Jones the opportunity to discuss a medication that can possibly target both issues. Bupropion is a medication that's indicated for the treatment of depression and has also been shown to be effective in improving Internet gaming disorder symptoms [5]. Hence, this may be an appropriate agent to consider for Ms. C. to improve her symptoms and her functioning. However, other medication options are limited, given that studies of the effectiveness of medications like escitalopram, methylphenidate, and atomoxetine, in the treatment of Internet gaming disorder, were not placebo controlled [5].

Similar to his treatment of gambling disorder, Dr. Jones should also discuss the benefit of a combined treatment approach with psychosocial interventions for Ms. C.'s Internet gaming disorder. Despite the limited studies, CBT has been shown to improve symptoms of Internet gaming disorder when administered alone or in tandem with bupropion. A combination of CBT and bupropion, in particular, was shown to be more effective than bupropion alone and may result in a better treatment outcome for Ms. C. In his approach to adolescent patients with Internet gaming disorder, Dr. Jones may also wish to consider family-based treatments, which are effective in treating SUDs in adolescents, but more research on their effectiveness for Internet gaming disorder is needed [5].

## Hypersexual Disorder

Mr. R. presents with hypersexual urges and behaviors consistent with hypersexual disorder, as well as chronic anxiety likely secondary to his generalized anxiety disorder. His motivation to treat his sexual behaviors stems from the professional difficulties they have caused him, which is a common reason patients with this condition seek help [9]. Dr. Jones can discuss the medication options listed in Table 11.3, which have been shown to improve symptoms of both hypersexual disorder and common psychiatric comorbidities. In his approach to Mr. R.'s case, Dr. Jones may wish to consider SSRIs, which are used in the treatment of several anxiety disorders, including generalized anxiety disorder, and have been shown to effectively reduce hypersexual disorder symptoms [9]. In particular, he may wish to offer citalopram, which has been shown to improve masturbation frequency and pornography use in men, and may also help with anxiety. Other SSRIs to consider that have been shown to improve symptoms of hypersexual disorder, include fluoxetine, sertraline, and paroxetine. If Mr. R.'s hypersexual disorder symptoms show only partial improvement to SSRIs, Dr. Jones may also wish to consider adding naltrexone. This opioid antagonist may improve symptoms of hypersexual disorder when used alone or in combination with SSRIs and may be particularly beneficial for patients with co-occurring alcohol or opioid use disorders. Topiramate, on the other hand, which is an antiepileptic medication, may be beneficial for patients with comorbid alcohol use disorder, binge eating, or kleptomania. Lastly, in his approach to patients with comorbid bipolar disorder or schizophrenia, Dr. Jones could consider mood

**Table 11.3** Preferred pharmacologic agents for hypersexual disorder based on psychiatric comorbidities

| Pharmacologic agent(s) | Psychiatric comorbidities targeted | | |
|---|---|---|---|
| Selective serotonin reuptake inhibitors (citalopram, sertraline, paroxetine, fluoxetine) | Mood disorders other than bipolar spectrum disorders | Anxiety disorders (generalized anxiety disorder, social anxiety disorder, etc.) | – |
| Topiramate | Alcohol use disorder | Binge eating | Kleptomania |
| Mood stabilizers (lithium, valproate) | Bipolar disorder or bipolar spectrum disorders | Schizophrenia | – |
| Antipsychotics | Schizophrenia | Bipolar disorder or bipolar spectrum disorders | – |
| Naltrexone | Alcohol use disorder | Opioid use disorder | – |

stabilizers (i.e., lithium and valproate) or antipsychotics. However, he would need to exercise caution when choosing an antipsychotic, as certain agents such as aripiprazole can actually induce hypersexual symptoms [9].

In addition to an appropriate pharmacologic agent, Dr. Jones should discuss with Mr. R. the benefit of combination treatment, as discussed in the previous cases, including either CBT, referrals for self-help groups, or both [9].

## Conclusion

Controversy may continue about whether behavioral addictions should be recognized as mental disorders and how to categorize them, but the clinical cases in this chapter highlight the negative outcomes associated with these conditions when left untreated. Given the high rates of comorbid psychiatric disorders among gaming disorder, Internet gaming disorder, and hypersexual disorder, it is important for mental health providers to screen for other psychiatric symptoms when assessing patients with these conditions, as well as screen for problematic behaviors in patients presenting with various psychiatric complaints. A thorough assessment can subsequently guide medication selection to target the symptoms of both the behavioral addiction and any psychiatric comorbidities, which can be administered in tandem with psychosocial interventions.

### Key Points

- Gambling disorder, Internet gaming disorder, and hypersexual disorder can negatively impact patients' personal and professional lives, resulting in personal distress, and have been associated with high rates of comorbid psychiatric disorders.
- Combination treatment with available pharmacologic and psychosocial interventions has shown promise in improving the symptoms of these conditions.
- A comprehensive assessment of patients that screens for problematic behaviors and other psychiatric symptoms can inform the selection of optimal medications to target both behavioral addictions and their psychiatric comorbidities.

## References

1. Yau YH, Potenza MN. Gambling disorder and other behavioral addictions: recognition and treatment. Harv Rev Psychiatry. 2015;23(2):134–46.
2. Potenza MN, Balodis IM, Derevensky J, Grant JE, Petry NM, Verdejo-Garcia A, Yip SW. Gambling disorder. Nat Rev Dis Primers. 2019;5:51–1.
3. Ford M, Håkansson A. Problem gambling, associations with comorbid health conditions, substance use, and behavioural addictions: opportunities for pathways to treatment. PLoS One. 2020;15(1):e0227644. https://doi.org/10.1371/journal.pone.0227644.

4. Jo YS, Bhang SY, Choi JS, Lee HK, Lee SY, Kweon YS. Clinical characteristics of diagnosis for internet gaming disorder: comparison of DSM-5 IGD and ICD-11 GD diagnosis. J Clin Med. 2019;8(7):945. https://doi.org/10.3390/jcm8070945.
5. Zajac K, Ginley MK, Chang R, Petry NM. Treatments for internet gaming disorder and internet addiction: a systematic review. Psychol Addict Behav. 2017;31(8):979–94. https://doi.org/10.1037/adb0000315.
6. Saunders JB, et al. Gaming disorder: its delineation as an important condition for diagnosis, management, and prevention. J Behav Addict. 2017;6:271–9.
7. Burleigh TL, Griffiths MD, Sumich A, Stavropoulos V, Kuss DJ. A systematic review of the co-occurrence of Gaming Disorder and other potentially addictive behaviors. Curr Addict Rep. 2019;6:383–401.
8. Grubbs JB, Hoagland KC, Lee BN, Grant JT, Davison PM, Reid R, Kraus SW. Sexual addiction 25 years on: a systematic and methodological review of empirical literature and an agenda for future research. Clin Psychol Rev. 2020;82:101925.
9. Malandain L, Blanc JV, Ferreri F, Thibaut F. Pharmacotherapy of sexual addiction. Curr Psychiatry Rep. 2020;22:1–8.
10. Petry NM, Stinson FS, Grant BF. Comorbidity of DSM-IV pathological gambling and other psychiatric disorders: results from the National Epidemiologic Survey on Alcohol and Related Conditions. J Clin Psychiatry. 2005;66(5):564–74.
11. González-Bueno V, Santamaría JJ, Fernández D, Merino L, Montero E, Ribas J. Association between internet gaming disorder or pathological video-game use and comorbid psychopathology: a comprehensive review. Int J Environ Res Public Health. 2018;15(4):668.

# Co-occurring Substance Use Disorders and Mental Illness

# 12

Jonathan D. Avery and David Hankins

Only about 17% of individuals who need substance use treatment actually receive it [11]. The barriers that prevent those with substance use disorders from seeking care are both individual (e.g., shame, lack of insight, personal finances) and structural (e.g., lack of providers, stigma, high costs). These same barriers exist for those who need help for other mental health problems, compounding the difficulties that individuals who have both a substance use disorder and another mental illness can experience in seeking care [8]. In the United States alone, nine million people experiencing mental illness also have a co-occurring substance use disorder (SUD), and nearly half of them receive treatment for neither [11]. In this chapter, we discuss medication treatment for individuals with co-occurring disorders (CODs), with a particular focus on patients for whom medication would be indicated both for a mental illness and for a SUD.

Rates of all forms of substance use are higher in those with a co-occurring mental illness. Substance use in this population appears to be correlated with severity of mental illness, with those with more severe forms of mental illness the most likely to use substances. In 2018, 16% of adults without mental illness used any illicit drug in the United States, compared to 37% of adults with any mental illness and 49% of those with a serious mental illness (one that substantially limited one or more major life activities). Given the opioid crisis, it is particularly notable that those with serious mental illness use opioids at over five times the rate of those without mental illness, with 14.6% past year use compared to 2.6% [11]. Only 25% of adults with both opioid use disorder and another mental illness receive treatment for both [7]. The differences with alcohol are less stark but still statistically significant; 25% of

J. D. Avery · D. Hankins (✉)
Weill Cornell Medicine, NewYork–Presbyterian Hospital, New York, NY, USA
e-mail: joa9070@med.cornell.edu; dgh7001@med.cornell.edu



J. D. Avery, D. Hankins (eds.), *Addiction Medicine*, Psychiatry Update 2,
https://doi.org/10.1007/978-3-030-86430-9_12

those without mental illness engaged in binge alcohol consumption in the past month, compared to 32% of those with serious mental illness [7].

The consequences of untreated CODs have been consistently demonstrated. Among individuals with mental illness, all-cause mortality is two to three times higher in those with a COD than those without [6]. Individuals with co-occurring major depression and a SUD have more severe depressive episodes more often, more suicide attempts, and greater risk of experiencing other mental illnesses compared to those who have major depression without a SUD [4]. Patients with schizophrenia and a COD have two to three times more psychiatric hospitalizations than those with schizophrenia alone [9]. Taken together, these studies and many others emphasize the importance of treating both mental illnesses and CODs.

Psychosocial interventions (such as 12-step programs and brief interventions at office visits) are an important component of treatment for SUDs. Utilizing only psychosocial interventions, however, misses an opportunity for the use of a range of safe and effective medication treatments for SUDs. This can happen even in cases where both patient and psychiatrist feel comfortable with medication treatment for a mental illness; barriers often cited to the initiation of such treatment include lab monitoring requirements, concern for risk of diversion, and perceived lack of time [1].

The three substance use disorders for which there is the strongest evidence in support of pharmacology as a key treatment modality are alcohol, nicotine, and opioid use. Note that the *Diagnostic and Statistical Manual of Mental Disorders, Fifth Edition* (DSM-5) was released before the widespread use of non-tobacco nicotine products, such as electronic cigarettes; in this chapter we retain the DSM-5 terminology of tobacco use disorder. These three substances represent, along with cannabis, the most commonly used and abused substances in the United States [11]. Table 12.1 highlights some of the evidence-based medication treatments for alcohol, opioid, and tobacco use disorders [2].

The clinical case in this chapter will illustrate how a comprehensive approach to individuals with CODs can include the use of medications for both substance use disorders and a range of other psychiatric diagnoses.

## Clinical Case

Dr. Walker is a psychiatry resident early in her third year of training, working at an outpatient clinic in a large urban area. Dr. Walker's schedule for the day includes three patients she has met for the first time recently but does not yet know well. Her first patient, Deborah, is a 42-year-old woman with a history of schizophrenia, who has been treated in the outpatient clinic for over a decade. She has tried several antipsychotics during that time but is now stable on risperidone. Deborah reports that she has been binge drinking recently up to two six packs of beer nightly, although on some days she does not drink at all. She says this has been her pattern of alcohol consumption for many years and is unsure if the frequency or amount of her alcohol use has changed recently. She did not discuss this at their first

**Table 12.1** Psychopharmacology for substance use disorders, with average doses

| Alcohol use disorder | Opioid use disorder | Tobacco use disorder |
|---|---|---|
| Naltrexone (ReVia)<br>50 mg PO QD | Buprenorphine[a]<br>(Suboxone)<br>8–16 mg SL QD | Varenicline (Chantix)<br>1 mg PO BID |
| Naltrexone (Vivitrol)<br>380 mg IM monthly | Methadone (Dolophine, Methadose)<br>60–120 mg PO QD | Bupropion (Wellbutrin, Zyban)<br>150 mg PO BID of sustained release, or<br>300 mg PO QD of extended release |
| Acamprosate (Campral)<br>666 mg PO TID | Naltrexone (ReVia)<br>50 mg PO QD | Nicotine replacement therapies |
| Disulfiram (Antabuse)<br>125–500 mg PO QD | Naltrexone (Vivitrol)<br>380 mg IM monthly | |
| Gabapentin (Neurontin)<br>600–2400 mg PO QD | | |
| Topiramate (Topamax)<br>75–150 mg PO BID | | |

Note. *PO* orally, *QD* once daily, *TID* three times daily, *SL* sublingual

[a]Usually combined with naloxone and available in several forms and preparations (film, tablet, implants)

appointment together a month ago and has never received any kind of alcohol-specific treatment.

Second on the schedule for the day is Kay, a 27-year-old woman with generally well-controlled bipolar I disorder. Kay has had severe manic and depressive episodes in the past, requiring hospitalization five times. Kay began using oxycodone ten months ago after a back surgery and four months ago began injecting heroin. She is interested in stopping but is wary of treatment options given that her regimen of lithium and quetiapine already leaves her at times feeling in her words "overmedicated." Her lithium levels have been erratic over the past several months despite no change in her dose.

Dr. Walker's final patient, Zack, is a 53-year-old man who has been in treatment for major depressive disorder and without full remission of symptoms on sertraline for the past five months. Dr. Walker has used a brief motivational approach at each visit to discuss Zack's cigarette smoking, which is currently at 30 cigarettes per day.

After seeing these patients, Dr. Walker prepares to discuss the cases with her attending and considers how she might be able to manage these individuals' CODs.

## Discussion

Dr. Walker's patients for the day present with three of the most common substance use disorders, in the setting of existing psychiatric diagnoses which are likely the primary reason that they are coming to see a psychiatrist. Given the amount that must be covered in a single psychiatric appointment, the temptation to focus solely on the primary psychiatric issue and thus neglect any CODs is understandable. However, given the beneficial effects that can come from stopping these substances in terms of patients' physical and mental health, taking some time at each visit to review current substance use and available medication treatment options can pay substantial dividends.

Some of the hesitation in discussing medication treatments for CODs with patients likely emerges from provider mindsets about substance use disorders more broadly. Society at large and many individual providers have tended to view SUDs as primarily behavioral or a reflection of moral failing on the part of the patient and thus best addressed with psychosocial interventions [3]. An approach that combines psychosocial and pharmacologic interventions is likely to be more beneficial for patients, with a particular focus on medication treatments for the three substance use disorders highlighted in this chapter.

## Treatment

### Alcohol Use Disorder

Deborah's pattern of alcohol use warrants further discussion at her psychiatry appointments and would likely benefit from the initiation of medication treatment. One important consideration for Dr. Walker will be her assessment of Deborah's overall level of adherence to her prescribed schizophrenia regimen of oral risperidone. If Deborah has been adherent, Dr. Walker might consider the addition of any of the oral agents mentioned in Table 12.1. However, Dr. Walker should also consider and discuss with Deborah long-acting intramuscular naltrexone, which could help reduce pill burden and improve adherence in any patient, but particularly those with the risk factors for cognitive impairment that come from both problematic alcohol use and from schizophrenia. Given Deborah's history of schizophrenia, for which long-acting injectable formulations are one of the mainstays of treatment, Dr. Walker might be able to initiate the conversation by exploring Deborah's history with injections, if any, and her thoughts on oral versus injectable medications. Deborah's reported pattern of binge alcohol use with days of abstinence may also make her a candidate for the "Sinclair method" of oral naltrexone use, in which naltrexone is taken only on days when a patient is drinking, to reduce the amount of alcohol consumed [10]. Baseline laboratory tests to measure liver and kidney function could help narrow the list of acceptable options; acamprosate can cause kidney damage, and naltrexone and disulfiram are implicated in liver disease (Table 12.2).

### Opioid Use Disorder

Kay presents to Dr. Walker with the relatively recent onset of a COD, in this case use of prescription painkillers and heroin, and a clearly stated desire to stop using, creating a unique opportunity to collaboratively pursue medication-assisted treatment. The ambivalence she expressed about being on another medication is worth further exploration, so that Dr. Walker can understand if this is related to forgetting to take her medications, side effects, cost, or any number of other potential factors.

**Table 12.2** Advantages and contraindications to medications for alcohol use disorder

| Medication | Advantages | Contraindications |
|---|---|---|
| Naltrexone | Oral or injectable formulations<br>Oral form can be taken daily or only on days when patient is drinking<br>Strong evidence base | Liver disease<br>Active opioid use |
| Acamprosate | Useful for those patients with liver damage (renally cleared)<br>Typically very well tolerated | Kidney disease |
| Disulfiram | Useful particularly for highly motivated patients | Concurrent alcohol use<br>Coadministration with any of several antibiotics, and a few rarer drugs can compound the "disulfiram reaction" if taken with alcohol<br>Severe liver or heart disease |
| Gabapentin | Can treat anxiety disorders | None |
| Topiramate | Mood stabilizing properties | None |

The variation in her lithium level could suggest some degree of nonadherence, particularly if other causes have been excluded.

Dr. Walker could propose the main treatment options for opioid use disorder to Kay: methadone, buprenorphine, or the long-acting intramuscular formulation of naltrexone. Methadone would require referral to a specialty clinic and, if initiated, attention to a number of potentially serious drug-drug interactions including for several commonly used psychiatric medications (benzodiazepines and some antidepressants can raise methadone levels, while carbamazepine among others can lower levels). Office inductions onto buprenorphine are becoming more widespread as provider training in its use is growing. Since Dr. Walker has completed buprenorphine training, initiating buprenorphine might be a particularly appealing option to take advantage of Kay's expressed desire to stop using opioids. Buprenorphine has considerably fewer clinically significant drug-drug interactions than methadone as well, potentially making the path forward easier if Kay were to need adjustments to the medication regimen for her bipolar I disorder in the future. Long-acting intramuscular naltrexone is also an option in this case, especially if an injectable formulation is sought either for patient preference or to improve adherence. However since Kay's opioid use originated from a surgery, methadone or buprenorphine may be preferable to long-acting naltrexone in this case due to their analgesic effects.

## Tobacco Use Disorder

Zack, who has both major depressive disorder and tobacco use disorder, also has many medication treatments available to treat his COD. In this case, one medication is indicated for both diagnoses: bupropion. Dr. Walker could discuss with Zack whether he has ever tried bupropion before or if it was previously stopped should explore dosing (to ensure a high enough treatment dose was attempted), side effects, and duration of the trial. This is a particularly attractive option since Zack's depression has not achieved remission with sertraline; bupropion could be considered for either a new monotherapy or as an adjunctive agent for sertraline [5].

In addition to bupropion, other medication options for the management of Zack's tobacco use disorder include nicotine replacement therapy (available in a variety of delivery systems including patches, gum, lozenges, inhalers, and others) and varenicline.

Although this would not be the case for Zack, it is important to keep in mind for other patients that by-products from tobacco smoke induce cytochrome P450 (CYP) 1A2, lowering the serum drug levels for antipsychotics including haloperidol, olanzapine, and clozapine. This induction does not happen with nicotine-only products. Thus if a patient is abstinent from tobacco for a time (including with the aid of nicotine replacement therapy) and then resumes smoking, this can lead to a rapid emergence of psychotic symptoms. Given high rates of relapse back to nicotine, patients with tobacco use disorder as a COD should continue to be asked about their tobacco use even after a period of abstinence.

## Conclusion

The high number of patients with mental illness who also have a COD should prompt mental health providers to carefully screen for substance use disorders and to consider pharmacologic treatments for their patients' CODs. Each medication comes with its own profile of advantages and risks, giving providers options to tailor treatments to patients' unique needs and preferences.

### Key Points

- Individuals with co-occurring disorders (CODs) are at risk of having their substance use disorder (SUD) go untreated even if they are in psychiatric care.
- A range of effective psychopharmacologic options are available to treat alcohol, opioid, and tobacco use disorders, which are three of the most common substance use disorders.
- Medication treatments for CODs typically interact minimally with pharmacologic agents for other psychiatric diagnoses or have drug-drug interactions that can be considered and adapted to.

## References

1. Albright J, et al. Psychiatrist characteristics that influence use of buprenorphine medication-assisted treatment. J Addiction Med. 2010;4(4):197–203. https://doi.org/10.1097/ADM.0b013e3181c816f3.

2. Avery JD. Pharmacological interventions. In: Avery JD, Barnhill JW, editors. Co-occurring mental illness and substance use disorders: a guide to diagnosis and treatment. Arlington: Am Psychiatric Assoc Publishing; 2018. p. 185–98.
3. Avery JJ, et al. Physicians' and attorneys' beliefs and attitudes related to the brain disease model of addiction. American J Addictions. 2020;29(4):305–12. https://doi.org/10.1111/ajad.13023.
4. Blanco C, et al. Differences among major depressive disorder with and without co-occurring substance use disorders and substance-induced depressive disorder: results from the National Epidemiologic Survey on Alcohol and Related Conditions. J Clin Psych. 2012;73(6):865–73. https://doi.org/10.4088/JCP.10m06673.
5. DeBattista C, et al. A prospective trial of bupropion SR augmentation of partial and non-responders to serotonergic antidepressants. J Clin Psychopharmacol. 2003;23(1):27–30.
6. Hjorthøj C, et al. Association between alcohol and substance use disorders and all-cause and cause-specific mortality in schizophrenia, bipolar disorder, and unipolar depression: a nation-wide, prospective, register-based study. Lancet Psychiatry. 2015;2(9):801–8. https://doi.org/10.1016/S2215-0366(15)00207-2.
7. Jones CM, McCance-Katz EF. Co-occurring substance use and mental disorders among adults with opioid use disorder. Drug Alcohol Depend. 2019;197:78–82. https://doi.org/10.1016/j.drugalcdep.2018.12.030.
8. Priester, et al. Treatment access barriers and disparities among individuals with co-occurring mental health and substance use disorders: an integrative literature review. J Substance Abuse Treatment. 2016;61:47–59. https://doi.org/10.1016/j.jsat.2015.09.006.
9. Schmidt LM, Hesse M, Lykke J. The impact of substance use disorders on the course of schizophrenia—a 15-year follow-up study: dual diagnosis over 15 years. Schizophr Res. 2011;130(1–3):228–33. https://doi.org/10.1016/j.schres.2011.04.011.
10. Sinclair JD. Evidence about the use of naltrexone and for different ways of using it in the treatment of alcoholism. Alcohol Alcohol. 2001;36(1):2–10. https://doi.org/10.1093/alcalc/36.1.2.
11. Substance Abuse and Mental Health Services Administration. Key substance use and mental health indicators in the United States: Results from the 2018 National Survey on Drug Use and Health (HHS Publication No. PEP19-5068, NSDUH Series H-54). Rockville, MD: Center for Behavioral Health Statistics and Quality, Substance Abuse and Mental Health Services Administration; 2019. Retrieved from https://www.samhsa.gov/data/.

# Index




J. D. Avery, D. Hankins (eds.), *Addiction Medicine*, Psychiatry Update 2,
https://doi.org/10.1007/978-3-030-86430-9

MIX
Papier aus verantwortungsvollen Quellen
Paper from responsible sources
FSC® C105338

If you have any concerns about our products,
you can contact us on
**ProductSafety@springernature.com**

In case Publisher is established outside the EU,
the EU authorized representative is:
**Springer Nature Customer Service Center GmbH**
**Europaplatz 3, 69115 Heidelberg, Germany**

Printed by Libri Plureos GmbH
in Hamburg, Germany